Va Va Voom

As a Registered Nutritional Therapist, Jackie Lynch is passionate about helping people achieve optimal health through good food. Jackie believes that nutritious food should be delicious and enjoyable and, as the founder of the WellWellWell clinic in London, this principle is at the heart of the nutrition advice and guidance she gives. *Va Va Voom* was inspired by people Jackie sees in her clinic who struggle with low energy and need practical and accessible food solutions to make a real difference to their everyday life.

Jackie writes regular nutrition features in the national press and on popular wellbeing websites. She also appears as a guest expert on television and radio lifestyle programmes, including Channel 4's *Superfoods*. Jackie is the author of *The Right Bite*, a one-stop guide to smart food and drink choices on the go. She writes a regular blog on her website www.well-well-well.co.uk or you can follow her on Facebook and Twitter at @WellWellWellUK.

Va Va Voom

THE 10-DAY ENERGY DIET

JACKIE LYNCH

Copyright © 2017 Jackie Lynch

The right of Jackie Lynch to be identified as the Author of the Work has been asserted by her in accordance with the Copyright, Designs and Patents Act 1988.

First published in 2017
by HEADLINE HOME
An imprint of HEADLINE PUBLISHING GROUP

1

Apart from any use permitted under UK copyright law, this publication may only be reproduced, stored, or transmitted, in any form, or by any means, with prior permission in writing of the publishers or, in the case of reprographic production, in accordance with the terms of licences issued by the Copyright Licensing Agency.

Every effort has been made to fulfil requirements with regard to reproducing copyright material. The author and publisher will be glad to rectify any omissions at the earliest opportunity.

Illustrations © light_s/Shutterstock

Cataloguing in Publication Data is available from the British Library

Trade Paperback ISBN 978 1 4722 5379 8

Typeset in Chaparral Pro by Palimpsest Book Production Limited, Falkirk, Stirlingshire

Printed and bound in Great Britain by Clays Ltd, St Ives plc

Headline's policy is to use papers that are natural, renewable and recyclable products and made from wood grown in sustainable forests. The logging and manufacturing processes are expected to conform to the environmental regulations of the country of origin.

HEADLINE PUBLISHING GROUP
An Hachette UK Company
Carmelite House
50 Victoria Embankment
London
EC4Y 0DZ

www.headline.co.uk
www.hachette.co.uk

Dad, this one's for you! With my love and thanks
for a lifetime of support and encouragement.
And for all the laughs we've shared.

Contents

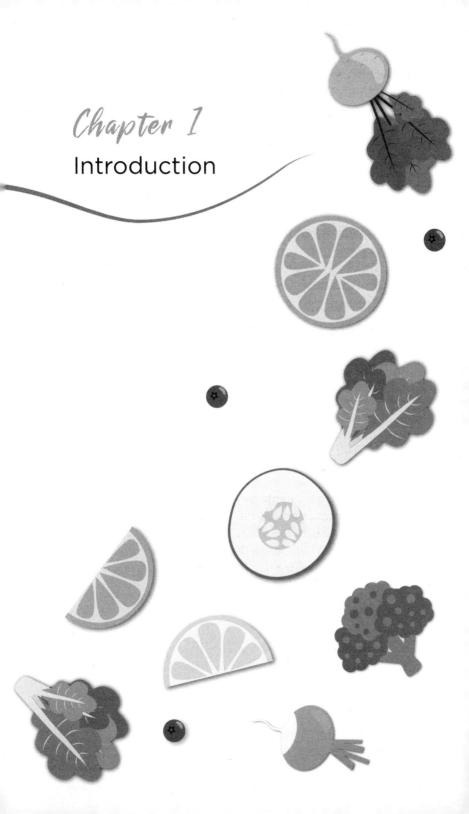

Chapter 1
Introduction

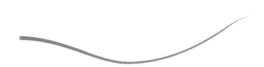

Have you lost your Va Va Voom? Are you TATT? Doctors use this shorthand for something they come across every single day: 'Tired All the Time' is when a patient continually complains of fatigue, yet there's no underlying medical condition.

In my nutrition clinic I constantly hear people say, 'It must be my age' as the reason for their lack of energy. If this sounds familiar, it's definitely time to take action. Whether you're 29 or 69, it's far more likely that your diet and lifestyle are the main culprits and a few simple changes and new habits can make a world of difference to how you feel.

I've written this book for all of you who don't want to take your lack of energy lying down! It's a simple, practical diet and lifestyle plan to help you rediscover your Va Va Voom in just 10 days.

WHO IS THIS BOOK FOR?

Whether you're feeling generally tired, are prone to energy highs and lows or just feel that you've lost a bit of zip, the Va Va Voom plan is designed to help you regain and sustain your physical and mental energy. It's suitable for anyone who thinks they'd benefit from a bit more energy in their life.

If you already know that your lack of energy is due to a diagnosed medical condition such as poor thyroid function, an autoimmune condition or a chronic illness such as cancer, kidney or cardiovas-cular disease, the Va Va Voom diet and lifestyle advice in this book may be very helpful in supporting your medical treatment. However, it's important to discuss any planned changes to your diet with your doctor before you embark on the 10-day plan to check that it's suitable for you.

If you feel unusually tired and your symptoms persist or are unrelieved by rest, it's advisable to see your doctor to rule out any underlying medical condition that may be contributing to a loss of energy before you try out the 10-day plan.

The Va Va Voom plan is not designed to be a weight-loss diet, but it's not unusual to lose a few pounds over the 10 days. This is because many of the foods and drinks which rob us of energy are also those that contribute to weight gain, and these will be eliminated during the programme.

HOW TO USE THIS BOOK

If you want to get cracking straight away you can skip to Chapter 5 and get started on the Va Va Voom plan as soon as you like. However, if you're keen to get the most out of the plan, then it's best to spend some time working through the next few chapters because they will help you identify the potential Va Va Voom issues that relate specifically to you. This will enable you to take a more personalised approach to the plan by focusing on the diet or lifestyle issues that are most relevant for you.

Where To Begin

Start out by reading the 'Energy Made Easy' section on pages 7–9 to help you understand the vital role that different nutrients play in this process. Simply ensuring that your diet contains plenty of these key nutrients will make it so much easier for your body to produce energy.

The Va Va Voom Quiz

The Va Va Voom quiz in Chapter 2 will help you identify the weak points in your energy production so that you can assess whether your loss of Va Va Voom might be related to nutrient deficiency, blood sugar management, lifestyle factors or a possible food sensitivity.

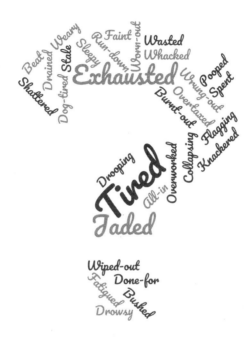

There are many different types of energy, which is why there are many different words to describe tiredness and fatigue. Which words best describe how you feel?

Va Va Voom Boosters and Robbers

Once you've identified some possible contributors to your loss of energy, Chapters 3 and 4 will provide targeted information on a whole series of food and lifestyle factors that can either boost or rob your energy. You can either read through them all or you can focus on the ones identified as the most likely issues for you in the Va Va Voom quiz. The information in these sections will enable you to include the most relevant foods for you in your 10-day plan and it will also provide some practical advice to help you avoid any lurking energy-robbing pitfalls.

The 10-Day Va Va Voom Plan

The Va Va Voom plan is modular and builds up slowly, allowing a gentle transition between the different phases so that it isn't too much of a shock to the system. There are two versions of the plan, The Energiser and The Super-Boost, so that you can select the one which is more appropriate for you. They both follow the same principles but The Energiser moves at a slower pace and has longer transition phases. Each plan consists of a diet and a wellbeing section and it's important to commit to both elements if you want to regain your Va Va Voom.

The Va Va Voom Maintenance Plan

Once you've completed your 10-day Va Va Voom plan, you can move on to the Maintenance Plan. This plan will help you retain the energy-boosting habits you've acquired over the 10 days and it's full of helpful advice so that you can create your own sustainable Va Va Voom diet and lifestyle as you move forward. It takes a practical and flexible approach that's easy to fit into your schedule, allowing for social occasions and the odd treat without undoing all your good work.

Va Va Voom Recipes

The Va Va Voom recipe section provides a series of quick and easy recipes for all but the most basic of the suggested meals in the plan. You can use these to get you started or adapt them as you choose. It's absolutely fine to use your own recipes and meal ideas if you prefer, you simply need to make sure that you're respecting the Va Va Voom ingredients and portion guidelines for each stage of the plan.

ENERGY MADE EASY

Why Do I Need Energy?

You may think that energy is all about being able to run for the bus, juggle work and family life or party all night, but that's just a very small part of why we need energy. In fact, every cell in our body requires energy to function properly.

Our brain is totally reliant on energy and if the brain cells aren't properly fuelled, loss of motivation, poor concentration, brain fog and confusion can occur. Without energy, our muscles can't function properly, and that includes the heart, which is one of our biggest muscles. When our muscles are starved of energy, it can lead to cramping and pain. Our immune cells use energy to fight infection and keep us healthy. We need energy to transport nutrients around the body and to absorb them into our cells. The entire reproductive process relies on energy for egg production and fertilisation. There's even a special energy store in sperm cells to maximise motility.

As our energy levels start to drop, any of these essential systems can be disrupted, which means that a lack of energy could be at the heart of a number of health concerns.

How Does the Body Produce Energy?

The energy-production process is a complex chain reaction in the body, a little bit like starting a car, and it relies on lots of different nutrients to activate each step. A deficiency in any one of these nutrients can make the process malfunction, which will cause our internal engine to stall.

It's All About Respiration

Respiration is more than just breathing (which is technically ventilation) – it refers to a whole sequence of reactions designed to convert our food into fuel. Most commonly, the body will use carbohydrate as a quick and easy energy source. Fat is converted to energy if you're low in carbohydrate or if there is a high demand for energy. Protein is usually a last resort and would mostly be broken down from body tissue if we're starved of other sources of energy.

During the respiration process, the food we eat reacts with oxygen to produce ATP (adenosine triphosphate) molecules that convert and store energy for the body to use when it needs it, a bit like charging and running a car battery. We need a constant supply of ATP to survive.

The Mitochondria – Your Personal Powerhouses

Respiration mostly takes place in small structures called mitochondria, which are found in each body cell in varying numbers. Healthy mitochondria are crucial to our energy levels, as they're responsible for producing about 90% of cellular energy. They combine fat, sugar or protein from our food with oxygen to produce energy.

Each mitochondrion contains its own DNA, which is essential to the function of the mitochondria. Mitochondrial DNA is different to the DNA responsible for our physical characteristics that is found in the nucleus of the cell. If your mitochondrial DNA is impaired, the energy-production process will be disrupted and your internal engine will start to misfire.

Unhealthy mitochondria will stop producing ATP molecules and start to consume them instead, using them as an energy source to keep going. Over time this may lead to cell damage or even cell death.

A number of things can affect the health of our mitochondria, including poor nutrition; exposure to toxins; ageing; stress; excessive exercise; disease and environmental factors.

The Chain Reaction

Glycolysis is where glucose (sugar) from our food is broken down through a series of steps to produce molecules called pyruvate. A few ATP energy molecules are produced as a by-product of this process.

The citric acid cycle is a complex process which starts with the conversion of the pyruvate into a compound called oxaloacetate which then leads to a cyclical series of reactions which produce some ATP molecules. During this cycle, hydrogen atoms are released into the mitochondrion, and these are vital for the next stage. If glucose is not available, other forms of carbohydrate, fat or protein can enter the citric acid cycle at various points through the process.

The electron transport chain is the stage that produces the most ATP energy molecules. The hydrogen atoms released during the citric acid cycle are converted into high energy electrons. These electrons pass along the electron transport chain, releasing energy as they go which is then converted into ATP.

38 ATP molecules can be produced by the entire respiration process of one glucose molecule.

How Does Nutrition Help Energy Production?

Each stage in the respiration process requires a number of key nutrients. These nutrients facilitate each conversion phase, from filling our fuel tank and igniting our engine to converting the fuel into energy. A deficiency in any of these nutrients can stall the entire energy-production process.

The citric acid cycle relies on certain B vitamins, magnesium, alpha-lipoic acid and iron to successfully complete a cycle.

The electron transport chain needs CoQ10, magnesium, zinc, copper, iron and vitamins B2, B3, C and K to function correctly.

Co-enzyme Q10 is a molecule found in the mitochondria. It's vital for energy production and is essential for the successful functioning of the electron transport chain. It works together with magnesium, carnitine and D-ribose (a form of sugar produced by the body) to help the mitochondria produce energy by kick-starting the whole process.

You can see how important the right nutrition is for the energy-production process so that your internal engine has a full tank that starts first time and runs smoothly throughout the day. All the elements of the 10-day plan are carefully designed to include plenty of these Va Va Voom-boosting nutrients.

So now it's over to you – you've read the theory and it's time to get started with the practice. Follow the plan carefully and make sure that you get your Va Va Voom back, once and for all!

Chapter 2

Why Have I Lost My Va Va Voom?

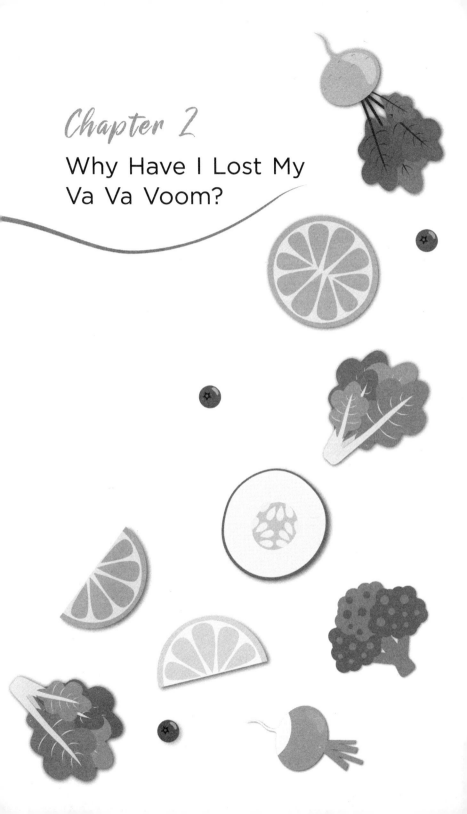

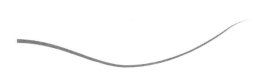

There are lots of possible factors that could be contributing to your loss of Va Va Voom. There's actually no formal diagnosis for fatigue; it's a subjective opinion about the way you're feeling and there are any number of reasons why you might be low in energy. It's always advisable to consult your doctor if symptoms persist or if you believe a medical condition could be at the root of your tiredness. However, in many cases, diet and lifestyle play a significant part in enhancing or depleting energy levels.

WHAT SORT OF ENERGY ARE YOU LACKING IN?

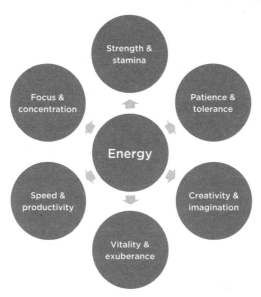

Energy manifests itself in different ways. Which of these types of energy do you feel most deficient in?

Understanding possible weak points in your energy production is an important first step in identifying the most appropriate diet and lifestyle solutions for you.

VA VA VOOM QUIZ

Try the Va Va Voom quiz to help you identify some of the factors that could be affecting your energy levels. Once you've completed each quiz, you can use the results to help you identify the energy boosters and energy robbers that may be most relevant to you.

Va Va Voom Quiz 1: Strength, Stamina and Concentration

Please answer the questions below, scoring 0 for never, 1 for occasionally, 2 for frequently or 3 for constantly

1. Do you feel tired and weak?
2. Is your skin paler than usual?
3. Do you bruise easily?
4. Do you have difficulty concentrating?
5. Do you experience headaches?
6. Do you experience palpitations?
7. Do you have aching or tingling muscles or joints?
8. Do you have a twitchy eyelid?
9. Do you feel unusually anxious, irritable or nervous?
10. Do you find it harder than usual to cope with stress or pressure?
11. Do you experience constipation?
12. Are you having difficulty getting to sleep?
13. Do you experience low mood?
14. Do you suffer from back or joint pain?

My Score out of 21 for questions 1–7

My Score out of 21 for questions 8–14

Scores

Questions 1–7 feature typical symptoms of a deficiency in iron or vitamin B12. Questions 8–14 feature symptoms that are characteristic of low levels of magnesium or vitamin D.

Score for Questions 1–7

0–3: Limited indication of any major concerns, but it's best to consult your doctor if any symptom is unusual for you.

4–11: You may wish to eat more foods that are rich in iron or vitamin B12 (see Chapter 3). If symptoms persist, consult your doctor for advice.

12–21: Multiple regular symptoms may indicate a deficiency in iron or vitamin B12. It would be advisable to consult your doctor for a diagnosis and advice about dietary supplements, if necessary. You may also benefit from eating more foods that are rich in iron or vitamin B12 (see Chapter 3).

Score for Questions 8–14

0–3: Limited indication of any major concerns, but it's best to consult your doctor if any symptom is unusual for you.

4–11: You may wish to eat more foods that are rich in magnesium (see Chapter 3). If symptoms persist, consult your doctor for advice about your vitamin D levels.

12–21: Multiple regular symptoms may indicate a deficiency in vitamin D or magnesium. It would be advisable to consult your doctor for a blood test and advice about dietary supplements, if necessary. You may also benefit from a diet and lifestyle approach to increase levels of these important nutrients (see Chapter 3).

Va Va Voom Quiz 2: Productivity, Creativity and Tolerance

Please answer the questions below, scoring 0 for never, 1 for occasionally, 2 for frequently or 3 for constantly

1. Do you often feel 'tired but wired'?
2. Have you experienced chronic stress or major stressful events in the past year?
3. Do you have abdominal fat that is difficult to shed?
4. Are you finding it harder than usual to manage stress?
5. Are you easily irritated or intolerant?
6. Do you struggle with concentration and focus?
7. Are you less creative than usual?
8. Do you find it hard to switch off?
9. Do you find it hard to work under pressure?
10. Do you find it hard to get going in the morning?
11. Do you feel you have the most energy after 6pm?
12. Do you find it difficult to throw off niggling colds and infections?
13. Do you drink more than 14 units of alcohol per week?*
14. Do you crave sugary or salty foods?
15. Is your motivation low?
16. Have you experienced a loss of libido?

*A bottle of 12% wine is about 9 units; a pint of 4% beer is about 2.5 units; a single 25ml spirit measure is 1 unit.

My Score out of 48 ( )

Scores

The symptoms outlined in this quiz are all characteristic of exposure to chronic stress, which can significantly deplete energy levels.

0–9: Limited indication of any major concerns but it's best to consult your doctor if any symptom is unusual for you.

10–27:   You may wish to focus on nutrients that help to regulate the body's response to stress (see Chapter 4). If symptoms persist, consult your doctor for advice.

28–48:   Multiple regular symptoms suggest that your stress levels may have become excessive. It may be time to consider slowing down or changing your lifestyle. Focusing on stress-busting foods may help (see Chapter 4) but do consult your doctor to rule out any medical conditions.

Va Va Voom Quiz 3: Focus, Patience and Endurance

Please answer the questions below, scoring 0 for never, 1 for occasionally, 2 for frequently or 3 for constantly

1. Do you experience energy dips during the day?
2. Do you crave sugary foods or carbohydrate?
3. Do you rely on caffeine or sugar to keep you going?
4. Do you use alcohol to unwind after work?
5. Do you feel dizzy when you stand up?
6. Do you frequently skip breakfast because you don't feel like food in the morning?
7. Do you leave more than 4 hours between meals?
8. Do you get anxious or irritable when you don't eat regularly?
9. Do you find it difficult to lose weight?
10. Do you wake up 2–3 hours after going to sleep for no apparent reason?
11. Do you feel nervous, shaky or weak at times?

My Score out of 33

Scores

The symptoms outlined in this quiz are all characteristic of a blood sugar imbalance, which can cause energy peaks and troughs.

0–5: Limited indication of any major concerns but it's best to consult your doctor if any symptom is unusual for you.

6–19: You may benefit from a diet plan to help to balance your blood sugar (see Chapter 4). If symptoms persist, consult your doctor for advice.

20–33: Multiple regular symptoms suggest that you may have a blood sugar imbalance. It's advisable to consult your doctor to assess your blood glucose levels. It may also be beneficial to follow a blood sugar-balancing diet (see Chapter 4).

Va Va Voom Quiz 4: Vitality, Speed and Strength

Please answer the questions below, scoring 0 for never, 1 for occasionally, 2 for frequently or 3 for constantly

1.   Do you experience ongoing, unexplained fatigue?
2.   Do you experience abdominal bloating?
3.   Do you often feel sluggish or lethargic after eating?
4.   Is your tiredness unrelieved by rest?
5.   Do you get acid reflux?
6.   Do you experience diarrhoea and/or constipation?
7.   Do you experience abdominal pain or cramping?
8.   Do you often need to clear your throat?
9.   Do you have rhinitis, sinusitis or post-nasal drip?
10. Do you have dark circles under your eyes?
11. Do you experience 'brain fog'?
12. Do you get migraines?
13. Do you find it difficult to lose weight?
14. Do you struggle with skin issues such as psoriasis, eczema or dermatitis?

My Score out of 42

Scores

The symptoms outlined in this quiz are all characteristic of a food sensitivity which can affect your body in a variety of different ways.

0–9:   Limited indication of any major concerns, but if any symptom is unusual for you, it's best to speak to your doctor.

10–25: You may wish to keep a food diary to identify a possible link between your symptoms and the food that you're eating (see Chapter 4). If symptoms persist or are unusual for you, consult your doctor for advice.

26–42: Multiple regular symptoms may indicate some form of food sensitivity. Your first step should be to consult your doctor to rule out any medical condition and to discuss allergy testing. You may also benefit from an elimination diet (see Chapter 4) or a food intolerance test.

NEXT STEPS

The Va Va Voom quiz may have helped you to identify some diet and lifestyle factors that could be contributing to your lack of Va Va Voom. If you want to target these directly, you can move straight to the relevant sections in Chapters 3 and 4 to find out more. This could help you apply a more personalised approach to the 10-day plan.

However, there are a number of other factors that could also be at play. Taking your time to review all the different Va Va Voom boosters and robbers will ensure that you don't miss something that could be highly relevant to you.

Chapter 3
Va Va Voom Boosters

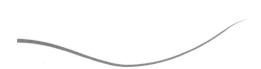

As we have seen, our energy production is a complex series of chain reactions which need the correct elements to operate in a specific sequence. It's a bit like starting and running a car – you'll need the fuel, the ignition, the spark plugs and engine oil to get moving and to stay moving. As with a car, our internal engine also needs the right support to work correctly, in this case a series of diet and lifestyle factors which play a vital role in producing and maintaining our energy. Making sure you have the right amounts of each of these Va Va Voom boosters in your diet and lifestyle will make a huge difference to your overall strength, stamina and vitality.

All of the elements in this chapter will play an essential role in supporting your energy production but you may want to pay particular attention to the diet and lifestyle factors that were highlighted as possible issues for you by the Va Va Voom quiz.

FUEL

Your body uses the macronutrients carbohydrate, fat and protein as fuel and combines them with oxygen to produce energy through a series of chain reactions. If you're not eating the correct balance of macronutrients, or you're not eating enough, you're at risk of running on empty.

CARBOHYDRATE

Carbohydrate is principally found in plants and there are three main types: sugar, starch and fibre. While 'carbs' is often used as a catch-all term for starchy food such as bread, potato or pasta, it's important to remember that fruit and vegetables also contain carbohydrates. Refined carbohydrate is produced when the fibre (as well as many micronutrients) has been stripped away from the grain during the manufacturing process, and therefore it can be broken down quickly by the body. White bread is an example of a refined carbohydrate. Complex carbohydrates such as wholegrains, pulses, vegetables and some fruits are more nutrient-dense, containing fibre, vitamins and minerals.

Why Do I Need Carbohydrate?

The single main purpose of sugar and starch is to provide glucose molecules which act as a quick and easy source of energy for the body. Fibre has a more complex role because it is non-digestible and therefore passes straight into the gut where it ferments, helping to increase levels of the beneficial bacteria required for healthy digestion and optimal immune function. Fibre also helps to regulate cholesterol levels.

DID YOU KNOW?

A bowl of oats every morning will do more than provide sustained energy. The soluble fibre in oats also plays a significant part in regulating cholesterol levels and promoting heart health.

How Does Carbohydrate Help My Energy Levels?

The brain is entirely dependent on glucose for energy but our whole internal engine responds quickly to glucose, therefore starch and sugar provide an incredibly rapid and powerful source of fuel. Fibre slows down the release of glucose into the body, which regulates blood sugar levels and provides a more sustained level of energy, putting your internal engine into cruising mode. This helps to avoid the energy peaks and troughs that come with the quick blast of energy from glucose.

DID YOU KNOW?

Potatoes and pasta contain a form of carbohydrate called resistant starch. This is reduced during cooking, but as the food cools down the levels can increase significantly – which is why cold potatoes or pasta can keep you going for longer.

Typical Symptoms of Carbohydrate Deficiency

- Low physical and mental energy
- Sugar cravings
- Constipation or loose stools
- Bloating or wind
- High cholesterol
- Poor immune function
- Blood sugar imbalance
- Headaches
- Flu-like symptoms

How Much Carbohydrate Do I Need?

Current advice is that we should be consuming at least 20g of fibre per day and this can be easily met by skewing the ratio of your 5-a-day towards vegetables instead of fruit. Starchy carbohydrate such as rice, bread, potatoes or pasta should make up around 25% of your plate at lunch and dinner and 50% of the meal should be vegetables – as wide a variety as possible. This will help to ensure the correct balance of fibre and starch, as well as support healthy digestion.

Fibre supplements should only be used under the guidance of a health professional as they may make your symptoms worse. If you are supplementing with fibre, it's important to build up the dosage slowly, as it can cause a bit of a shock to a sensitive digestion if you overdo it. You should drink plenty of water when taking fibre supplements to avoid constipation.

Why Might I Be Low in Carbohydrate?

- You're following a weight-loss diet which is strictly low-carb
- You're not eating enough fruit and vegetables
- You may be low in fibre if:
  - your diet is high in processed foods and ready meals rather than fibre-rich wholefoods
  - you tend to choose refined white flour products such as white bread, white rice or white pasta instead of fibre-rich wholemeal bread, brown rice or wholegrain pasta

3 Ways to Boost Your Carbohydrate Levels

1. Boost your fibre intake by swapping from white to brown foods; choose wholemeal bread, brown rice or wholegrain pasta.
2. Eat 5 portions of vegetables every day.
3. Eat more plant proteins, such as lentils, beans or chickpeas as these are also an excellent source of fibre.

FAT

There are three main natural forms of fat: saturated, monounsaturated and polyunsaturated, and the body needs all of them for a range of vital functions. Foods that contain fat will contain all three forms, but the ratio will vary. For example, red meat and dairy products tend to be higher in saturated fat and lower in unsaturated fats, and fish, nuts and seeds are usually higher in unsaturated fats and lower in saturated fat.

Why Do I Need Fat?

We need saturated fat to produce cholesterol, which is critical in the correct amount. Our sex hormones are synthesised from cholesterol and we also need it to produce the stress hormone cortisol, which regulates the 'fight or flight' response (see Chapter 4). Monounsaturated and polyunsaturated fats (which include the omega 3, 6 and 9 fats) promote heart health and the flexibility and fluidity of blood vessels. They support skin and hormone health and contribute to the optimum functioning of the nervous system. We need fat to absorb and store fat-soluble vitamins A, D, E and K.

How Does Fat Help My Energy Levels?

Fat is a premium source of fuel for the body, containing twice as much energy per gram as carbohydrate or protein. It's the ideal fuel for our spark plugs to convert into physical energy and will keep our engine running well for hours, as long as there isn't too much glucose for the body to use instead. The anti-inflammatory omega 3 fatty acids help to relieve the burden of chronic inflammation which significantly depletes our energy resources. Our brain has a high concentration of fat and depends on monounsaturated fats to optimise the blood flow and energy supply to the brain and to support the neurotransmitters which facilitate focus, concentration and learning.

Typical Symptoms of a Deficiency in Fat

- Dry, flaky or dull skin
- Small bumps on the back of your upper arms
- Low levels of vitamin D
- Neurological disorders
- Poor concentration or focus
- Impaired vision
- Low mental energy
- Menstrual disorders
- Vaginal dryness
- Stiff or aching joints
- Low mood
- Fatigue

How Much Fat Do I Need?

We need to be eating around 70g of total fat each day. Of this, saturated fat should make up about 20g for women and 30g for men with the rest consisting of mono and polyunsaturated fat. A 100g steak contains around 25g of saturated fat, 23g of monounsaturated fat and 2g of polyunsaturated fat. A 250ml glass of full-fat milk contains about 8g of saturated fat, 2.5g of monounsaturated fat and 0.1g of polyunsaturated fat. A 100g salmon steak contains about 3g of saturated fat, 6g of monounsaturated fat and 4g of polyunsaturated fat. A 25g handful of walnuts contains 1.5g of saturated fat, 3g of monounsaturated fat and 12g of polyunsaturated fats.

Fish oil is probably the most commonly used fatty acid supplement and it's advisable to choose pure fish oil rather than fish liver oil if you're looking to support omega 3 levels. Linseed oil is a suitable alternative for vegetarians. Evening primrose oil is a popular omega 6 supplement for women with PMS symptoms. Currently there is no formal recommended daily dose, so it's important to follow the manufacturer's instructions and not to exceed the dose on the bottle. Always check with your doctor before supplementing with fatty acids as they are a natural blood thinner and may interact with some medication.

DID YOU KNOW?

While polyunsaturated fats are generally very beneficial, too much omega 6 in the diet can activate inflammatory pathways. Manufacturers commonly use vegetable oils like sunflower or corn oil, which are high in omega 6, in processed foods such as biscuits, crackers, ready meals and fried foods, which has led to a significant increase in our consumption of omega 6. We should be aiming for a ratio of between 4:1 and 2:1 omega 6 to omega 3 but a Western diet is often somewhere between 8:1 and 25:1.

Why Might I Be Low in Fat?

- You consciously choose low-fat products such as skimmed milk and low-fat yoghurt or houmous
- High levels of omega 6 fatty acids in your diet can compromise the action of omega 3 in the body
- Unsaturated fats (such as omega 9 in olive oil) are unstable and can be denatured by high temperatures, which will affect your ability to absorb them
- High levels of artificial trans fats in the diet may compromise the absorption of omega 3 in the body. Trans fats are commonly found in fried fast food and processed foods to prolong shelf life

DID YOU KNOW?

Manufacturers often add extra sugar or salt to low-fat products to replace the flavour that has been stripped out along with the fat.

3 Ways to Boost Your Fat Levels

1. Opt for full-fat instead of low-fat products.
2. Snack on raw almonds, walnuts and pumpkin seeds instead of biscuits or chocolate.
3. Reduce your consumption of fried fast food and processed food as these can block the action of healthy fats.

PROTEIN

Protein is made up of building blocks called amino acids. Nine of these are essential amino acids which need to be acquired through the diet. The body is able to synthesise the remaining amino acids that we need.

Animal sources of protein, such as meat, fish and eggs contain all the essential amino acids in one easy package – they are 'complete' proteins. Most plant proteins, such as pulses, nuts or seeds contain some but not all the essential amino acids, which is why a good variety of protein is required if you're following a vegetarian diet. Quinoa and soya are examples of complete plant proteins.

Why Do I Need Protein?

The human body is built of protein and we'd grind to a complete halt without it. We need it for growth and repair of every element of our body, from bones and tissue to hair and nails. Every cell relies on protein to function. Proteins also help to regulate fluid balance and to transport nutrients around the body.

How Does Protein Help My Energy Levels?

As we have seen in Chapter 1, protein isn't the body's preferred source of energy, although certain amino acids can help to increase endurance (see Amino Acids on page 58). However, protein plays an important indirect role in supporting energy levels via its role in blood sugar management. It helps to buffer the impact of sugars by slowing down their release into the bloodstream.

Eating protein with every meal and snack will keep you going for longer and promote sustained energy throughout the day. If you're low in protein, you're more likely to experience energy dips.

Typical Symptoms of Low Dietary Protein

- Brittle nails
- Hair loss
- Sugar cravings
- Lack of muscle tone
- Slow recovery from injury
- Soft bones
- Energy dips
- Bad skin
- Insomnia
- Depression
- Lack of stamina
- Poor memory
- Loss of concentration and focus

DID YOU KNOW?

The branched-chain amino acids leucine, isoleucine and valine (found in meat, fish, whey and soya protein) are especially important for energy and endurance, which is why they are often found in sports supplements. However, excessive levels of individual amino acids can be highly disruptive to the body and this could have serious health implications. Food sources of protein are likely to be safer and more effective in supporting your performance goals.

How Much Protein Do I Need?

Current advice is for 55g per day for adult males and 45g per day for adult females, although this may vary depending on height, build, physical activity and health status. Including protein in some form with every meal and snack will help to ensure that blood sugar levels are maintained, promoting sustained energy and providing that Va Va Voom factor.

Why Might I Be Low in Protein?

- You're not eating protein with every meal
- Your diet is low in complete protein
- Incomplete protein digestion in the stomach can lead to impaired protein absorption in the intestines
- Liver or kidney dysfunction can disrupt protein absorption

3 Ways to Boost Your Protein Intake

1. Add a tablespoon of chopped nuts or seeds daily to your morning cereal, muesli or granola.
2. Swap your usual rice, pasta or potato for quinoa.

3. Avoid protein-poor evening meals such as pasta with tomato sauce or pesto – adding tuna or chicken will make it a far more sustaining meal.

IGNITION

A tankful of fuel is a great start but it needs to be activated if you want to get it going and this is where the ignition process comes in. CoQ_{10} and carnitine help to prepare the fuel for use, and magnesium is the key that starts the engine, kicking off the whole process of energy production. Without your ignition nutrients, you won't even get off the starting line.

COENZYME Q_{10} (CoQ_{10})

Coenzyme Q_{10}, commonly known as CoQ_{10} or ubiquinone, is similar to a vitamin and acts as a powerful antioxidant. It's synthesised by the body but it's also found in small amounts in food. The best food sources of CoQ_{10} are oily fish such as salmon, mackerel and sardines, although you can also find it in other foods such as nuts, seeds and spinach in smaller quantities.

Why Do I Need CoQ$_{10}$?

Every cell in our body needs CoQ_{10} to function properly. It supports the immune function and the cardiovascular system, improving circulation and protecting our body from the free radical damage which is a key risk factor for age-related chronic disease. CoQ_{10} enhances the supply of oxygen to body cells and tissues and has a powerful anti-ageing effect.

How Does CoQ$_{10}$ Help My Energy Levels?

CoQ_{10} plays a critical role in the electron transport chain by working with the amino acid L-carnitine to draw fuel from the food we eat and convert it into energy. Low levels of CoQ_{10} can lead to mitochondrial dysfunction over time, which is the equivalent of a reduced power supply or, in severe cases, a power cut in our body resulting in a state of extreme low energy or chronic fatigue.

Typical Symptoms of a Deficiency in CoQ10

- Physical and mental fatigue
- High blood pressure
- Muscle weakness
- Frequent colds or infections
- Joint pain
- Headaches or migraines
- Poor exercise performance
- Fibromyalgia
- Chronic Fatigue Syndrome
- Heart disease

DID YOU KNOW?

Opting for a supplement that combines CoQ_{10} with vitamin E not only helps to preserve the CoQ_{10}, it also offers double the protection. CoQ_{10} enhances the antioxidant properties of vitamin E and they work together to reduce the risk of chronic disease.

How Much CoQ_{10} Do I Need?

There isn't a recommended minimum dietary intake of CoQ_{10} but if you mostly feel healthy and energised, you're probably either making all you need or getting enough from your food. A 100g portion of sardines contains about 6mg; a handful of peanuts or 2 large handfuls of spinach contain about 0.5mg. CoQ_{10} levels in the body will drop as we age so supplementing may be advisable, but it's very important to check with your doctor first because CoQ_{10} supplements may interact with heart and thyroid, and certain other, medication. There's currently no established recommended dosage for CoQ_{10} supplements but they generally range from 50–200mg per day, depending on the product. Never exceed the recommended dosage on the bottle and check with a health professional before you start taking CoQ_{10} if you have any concerns.

DID YOU KNOW?

Taking a CoQ_{10} supplement with oily fish such as salmon or mackerel will enhance the absorption into the body, because CoQ_{10} is a fat-soluble compound.

Why Might I Be Low in CoQ_{10}?

- Our CoQ_{10} levels decline with age so if you're over 50 this may be a consideration
- Certain medications such as statins may inhibit the production of CoQ_{10} in the body
- Poor diet can deplete our CoQ_{10} levels, as well as making it difficult for the body to produce CoQ_{10}
- Decreased levels of CoQ_{10} have been observed with chronic health conditions such as diabetes, cancer and heart disease

3 Ways to Boost Your CoQ_{10} Levels

1. Consider taking a supplement if you're over 50, but always check with your doctor first to avoid any potential interaction with medication.
2. Make sure you have a balanced wholefoods diet so that you provide your body with the right foods to support your in-house production of CoQ_{10}.
3. Top yourself up with CoQ_{10} by eating oily fish such as salmon, mackerel and sardines at least 3 times per week.

CARNITINE

Carnitine is similar to an amino acid but its role is very different because it's not used for protein synthesis nor is it converted into a neurotransmitter. In fact, it's mainly involved in energy production. The body uses a combination of amino acids, vitamins and minerals to produce carnitine, although it can also be found in animal foods such as meat and fish.

Why Do I Need Carnitine?

Optimum levels of carnitine are important for fat metabolism, helping to limit fatty deposits in our organs and tissues. It keeps our cells healthy by preventing a build-up of toxins and it also supports muscle strength, endurance and sperm motility. Carnitine works in synergy with vitamins C and E to enhance their antioxidant effect and slow the ageing process.

How Does Carnitine Help My Energy Levels?

The main function of carnitine is to enable us to use our food as fuel. It transports fat into our cells so that it can be converted into energy for our muscles and tissues, increasing the body's use of fat as an energy source. A by-product of carnitine is acetyl-L-carnitine which also supports energy production by promoting carbohydrate metabolism and increasing the concentration of carnitine in body tissues.

Typical Symptoms of a Deficiency In Carnitine

- Muscle weakness or wastage
- Low energy
- Dizziness
- Chest pain
- Palpitations
- Irritability
- Confusion
- Decreased sperm motility
- Obesity

DID YOU KNOW?

L-carnitine is the active form of carnitine which is involved in the energy-production process. Supplementing with D-carnitine may reduce the effectiveness of L-carnitine.

How Much Carnitine Do I Need?

The body makes its own supply of carnitine from a combination of nutrients so there's no formal recommended dietary amount. If you want to top up your carnitine stocks through diet, the best sources tend to be animal foods. A 100g portion of beef contains up to 150mg of carnitine; a large glass of milk contains about 8mg and a slice of wholegrain bread contains around 0.1mg. Carnitine is available as a supplement, in the form of L-carnitine and dosages tend to range from 500–2000mg. Always check with your doctor before supplementing, because L-carnitine is a powerful nutrient which can interact with some medication, and never exceed the recommended dose.

Why Might I Be Low in Carnitine?

- A lack of vitamin C, B vitamins or iron in your diet can impair carnitine production
- A genetic disorder can reduce or prevent carnitine production
- People following a strict vegan diet have limited dietary sources of carnitine
- Carnitine can be excreted through sweat during intense exercise
- Chronic kidney or liver disease may reduce the body's ability to produce carnitine
- Certain medication may deplete carnitine levels

DID YOU KNOW?

L-carnitine can help to improve physical performance and endurance by enhancing the supply of energy to the muscles and supporting muscle recovery.

3 Ways to Boost Your Carnitine Levels

1. Make sure you eat plenty of vegetables and wholegrain foods as these are rich in vitamin C and B vitamins, essential for carnitine production.
2. Eat sources of animal protein such as meat and fish, or complete vegetable proteins such as soya or quinoa, as these contain the essential amino acids methionine and lysine which are used to make carnitine.
3. Limit your intake of alcohol and nicotine because these deplete B vitamins and vitamin C in the body, which may reduce carnitine production.

MAGNESIUM

You can find magnesium in lots of foods, but these are some of the top sources: leafy green vegetables such as spinach, watercress and kale; pumpkin and sunflower seeds; wholegrain foods such as brown rice, rye and quinoa; almonds and Brazil nuts.

Why Do I Need Magnesium?

Magnesium is the multi-tasker of the minerals: it's responsible for more than 300 essential chemical reactions throughout the body. It helps to regulate muscle function, underpins the nervous system and supports our response to stress. Magnesium is important for heart health because it regulates blood pressure and supports the nerve impulses and muscle contractions that are vital for a regular heart rhythm. It promotes peristalsis, the muscle action that moves stools through the bowel and therefore keeps our digestion regular. We also need magnesium for healthy bones and for the production of DNA.

How Does Magnesium Help My Energy Levels?

Magnesium starts your engine. If you're low in magnesium, you'll feel as if you're running on empty all the time because it's absolutely essential in the energy-production process. It maximises the production of ATP energy molecules in the citric acid cycle. In fact, magnesium is found within the ATP molecule itself. Without magnesium your internal engine would stall, because it activates the enzymes that spark the entire chain reaction of energy production in the body.

Typical Symptoms of a Magnesium Deficiency

- Constant fatigue or low energy
- Migraines
- Muscle weakness
- Muscle cramps, spasms or twitches
- Palpitations
- Anxiety
- Irritability
- Insomnia
- Constipation

DID YOU KNOW?

An Epsom salts (magnesium sulphate) bath is the perfect remedy after a stressful day. Add 2–3 handfuls to a bath and soak for 20 minutes (without using other bath products). The magnesium will be absorbed through the skin, relaxing the muscles, calming the nervous system and setting you up for a good night's sleep.

How Much Magnesium Do I Need?

Current advice suggests a minimum dietary intake of around 300mg per day for adults. That's not hard to achieve with a wholefoods diet – 2 tablespoons of sunflower seeds on your cereal provide about 80mg; a 100g portion of cooked spinach provides 100mg and a 100g portion of brown rice contains around 60mg. Supplementation should not exceed 400mg per day without the advice of a health professional. Magnesium can interact with certain medication so it's important to check with your doctor before taking any supplements.

DID YOU KNOW?

Regular calcium supplementation may be depleting your magnesium levels. High levels of calcium increase the body's need for magnesium because it cannot be effectively used or stored without magnesium.

Why Might I Be Low in Magnesium?

- You're not eating enough leafy green vegetables or wholegrains
- Chronic stress depletes magnesium in the body
- You're taking high-dose calcium supplements
- Certain medication, including some antibiotics and steroids, can deplete magnesium
- You may not be able to absorb magnesium from your food properly if you have suboptimal digestive function
- You're drinking too many fizzy drinks that contain phosphoric acid as this may impair magnesium absorption

3 Ways to Boost Your Magnesium Levels

1. Eat 2 handfuls of leafy green vegetables every day.
2. Make a point of opting for wholegrain foods such as wholemeal or rye bread, brown rice or wholegrain pasta.
3. Have an Epsom salts bath or foot bath once or twice a week.

SPARK PLUGS

The energy-production process relies on a series of catalyst nutrients that spark off the chain reaction that converts our fuel into energy. A lack of any of the nutrients in this section can disrupt the whole process, causing our internal engine to sputter or misfire, in the same way that if a car's spark plugs aren't working properly, it may still start but it will run very poorly.

B VITAMINS

B vitamins are a group of individual nutrients that work as a team to support a range of different functions in the body. A deficiency in one B vitamin is likely to indicate a deficiency in another. B vitamins are mostly found in wholegrain foods, vegetables and pulses or animal proteins, such as meat and eggs.

Why Do I Need B Vitamins?

Although they share a name, each B vitamin has a distinct supportive role within the body. They're categorised in a numbering system from 1–12, although some numbers no longer feature in the list because the nutrient was later discovered not to be a vitamin. Other B vitamins are better known by their full name.

B1 or thiamine supports cognitive function, learning capacity and memory.
B2 or riboflavin is needed for the formation of red blood cells and by the immune system for antibody production. It keeps the skin, hair and nails healthy and is vital for eye health. Low levels of B2 can inhibit the function of other B vitamins.
B3 or niacin helps to support brain function and the nervous system and enhances memory. It supports blood sugar balance, improves circulation and helps to lower cholesterol.
B5 or pantothenic acid is essential for a healthy nervous system and optimal immune function. It helps to reduce stress levels in

the body by supporting the production of adrenal hormones. It works in partnership with B2 to prevent anaemia.

B6 or pyridoxine has more jobs than almost any other single nutrient and it's important for both physical and mental health. It's vital for the healthy functioning of the brain and nervous system. It helps to balance sex hormones and relieve symptoms of PMS and can act as a natural anti-depressant by supporting the production of serotonin. It's also required for the absorption of B12.

B7 or biotin is especially important for cell growth which is why it's an important nutrient for children. It's essential for neurological development and is required for healthy skin and hair.

B9 or folate is essential in pregnancy for the neurological development of the foetus and remains essential throughout life for optimal functioning of the brain and nervous system. It is also required for the production of red blood cells.

B12 or cobalamin works in partnership with folate to form red blood cells and enhance the absorption of iron. It's vital for the correct functioning of the nervous system. It's required for the optimal digestion and absorption of foods and can help with memory and learning.

How Do B Vitamins Help My Energy Levels?

Acting as mini spark plugs, many of the B vitamins are important links in the conversion of carbohydrates, fats and proteins into energy during the process of respiration described in Chapter 1. B1 and B5 are essential to kick-start the citric acid cycle; without them, the entire energy-production process couldn't get started and your internal engine would begin to misfire. Vitamins B2 and B3 are required for the electron transport chain to function correctly.

The impact of Vitamins B6, B9 (folate) and B12 on energy production mainly comes from a different angle. These B vitamins are involved in the production of red blood cells, the transport of oxygen around the body and the optimal absorption of iron, ensuring our energy levels remain topped up at all times.

Typical Symptoms of a Deficiency in B Vitamins	
B1 (thiamine)	Irritability; poor memory and concentration; sore or weak muscles; fatigue; palpitations; digestive problems
B2 (riboflavin)	Sore or gritty sensation in the eyes; cracked lips or corners of the mouth; sensitivity to light; eczema or dermatitis; splitting nails and thinning hair; low energy
B3 (niacin)	Low energy; diarrhoea; low mood or depression; headaches or migraines; anxiety; irritability; insomnia; poor memory; loss of appetite
B5 (pantothenic acid)	Fatigue; nausea; tingling hands; burning feet; headaches; loss of motivation; anxiety or tension
B6 (pyridoxine)	Anaemia; headaches; nausea; water retention; nervousness or anxiety; dizziness; fatigue; inflammation of the mouth; flaky skin; sore tongue
B7 (biotin)	Dry skin, eczema or dermatitis; thinning hair; loss of appetite; muscular pain; cradle cap in infants; fatigue
B9 (folate)	Anaemia; sore tongue; fatigue; apathy; poor memory; low mood; elevated homocysteine, a risk factor for cardiovascular disease; impaired growth; prematurely greying hair; anxiety
B12 (cobalamin)	Exhaustion; poor memory; confusion; depression; dizziness; irritability or anxiety; pale skin; ringing in the ears; headaches; constipation; abnormal gait

How Much of Each B Vitamin Do I Need?

B vitamins can't be stored in the body, so they need to feature in your diet every day. While B vitamins are plentiful in a balanced diet, multiple lifestyle factors can affect their absorption in the body which means that supplement support may be relevant for you.

B1 (thiamine)	Adults require at least around 0.8mg of B1 each day from food. One slice of wholemeal bread provides around 0.12mg; 75g of peas contain roughly 0.18mg. Supplement intake should not exceed 100mg per day without the advice of a health professional.
B2 (riboflavin)	Adults require at least 1.1mg of riboflavin each day from food. One egg contains around 0.2mg and 100g of broccoli contains about 0.15mg. Supplement intake should not exceed 40mg per day without the advice of a health professional.
B3 (niacin)	Adults require at least 13mg of niacin each day from food. One slice of wholemeal bread contains 1.4mg; 100g of canned tuna contains around 12mg. Supplement intake should not exceed 17mg per day of B3 in the form of niacin or nicotinic acid or 500mg in the form of nicotinamide or niacinamide without the advice of a health professional.
B5 (pantothenic acid)	Adults require at least 3mg of pantothenic acid each day from food. 100g of lentils contain 0.31g; 4–5 medium strawberries contain roughly 0.09mg. Supplement intake should not exceed 200mg per day without the advice of a health professional.

B6 (pyridoxine)	Adults require at least 1.2mg of B6 each day from food. One green pepper (deseeded) contains around 0.37mg; one quarter of a 400g tin of kidney beans contain 0.1mg. Supplement intake should not exceed 200mg per day without the advice of a health professional.
B7 (biotin)	Biotin is only required in very small amounts by the body which is why it tends to be measured in micrograms (mcg) instead of milligrams (mg). There's no formal dietary recommendation as you should be able to get plenty from your diet. 100g of cauliflower contains around 1.5 mcg; a small glass of milk contains about 2 mcg. Supplement intake should not exceed 0.9mg per day without the advice of a health professional.
B9 (folate)	Folate (known as folic acid in supplement form) is also commonly measured in micrograms. Adults require at least 200mcg of folate each day from food. If you're pregnant or trying to conceive, you're advised to take 400mcg of folic each day, to help prevent birth defects. 100g of steamed broccoli contains around 72mcg; 30g of peanuts contain roughly 30mcg. Supplement intake should not exceed 1mg or 1000mcg per day without the advice of a health professional.
B12 (cobalamin)	Vitamin B12 is also measured in micrograms. Adults require at least 1.5mcg of B12 each day from food. A small 100g tin of sardines contains around 15mcg; 2 tablespoons of cottage cheese contain about 0.3mcg. Supplement intake should not exceed 2mg or 2000mcg per day without the advice of a health professional.

DID YOU KNOW?

Vitamin B12 is only naturally found in animal foods such as meat, fish and eggs; this means that people following a vegan diet can be at risk of a deficiency. Although certain cereals, some breads and yeast extract spreads are often fortified with B12, if you are a vegan it would be a smart move to check in with your doctor to assess your B12 levels from time to time, especially if you struggle with tiredness.

Why Might I Be Deficient in B Vitamins?

- You're not eating a wholefoods diet
- You follow a vegan diet
- Regular alcohol consumption: all B vitamins are depleted by alcohol
- You have a stressful lifestyle or you suffer from chronic stress: stress depletes B vitamins
- You boil your vegetables: up to 40% of B vitamins are lost by using this cooking method
- Certain B vitamins can be depleted by the oral contraceptive pill
- Poor nutrient absorption in the gut
- You have pernicious anaemia, an autoimmune condition which prevents the absorption of B12

DID YOU KNOW?

B vitamins are water soluble which means the B vitamin content of vegetables will be reduced by 30–40% if you're in the habit of boiling them, as the vitamins will leach into the water. Once you've strained them, you could literally be throwing a lot of B vitamins down the drain! Steaming your vegetables is a better way to maximise their nutritional value.

3 Ways to Boost Your B Vitamin Levels

1. Aim to eat 5 portions of a variety of vegetables every day.
2. Enhance your absorption of B vitamins by limiting your alcohol intake – the more alcohol-free days you can manage each week, the more B vitamins your body will be able to draw from your diet.
3. Buy a steamer for your vegetables and make sure you cook them lightly to preserve as many B vitamins as possible.

VITAMIN C

Vitamin C is a powerful antioxidant which is mostly found in vegetables, fruit and herbs. Top sources include green vegetables, peppers, kiwi fruit, papaya and parsley. Beware of orange juice: while freshly squeezed orange juice is a good source of vitamin C, the pasteurisation or heat treatment of the juice in many carton products may significantly reduce the levels of vitamin C.

Why Do I Need Vitamin C?

Vitamin C has multiple roles in the body. It supports immune function and helps to fight infection and promote wound healing. We need it for healthy bones, skin and blood vessels. It's a highly protective antioxidant which can help reduce the toxicity of heavy metals and pollution. We need vitamin C for the production of certain key hormones and to support the absorption of iron. It also helps to regulate the body's response to stress.

How Does Vitamin C Help My Energy Levels?

Low levels of vitamin C can leave you feeling weak and lethargic. It's a hugely important catalyst in the electron transport chain, which is the stage of respiration that produces the most energy molecules (see Chapter 1). We also need it to produce carnitine, the nutrient that kick-starts energy production in the mitochondria.

Typical Symptoms of Vitamin C Deficiency

- Frequent colds and infections
- Low energy
- Bleeding or soft gums
- Easy bruising
- Joint pain
- Poor skin
- Poor wound healing
- Scurvy

DID YOU KNOW?

Vegetables tend to be much higher in vitamin C than fruit, with a red pepper containing twice as much vitamin C as an orange, gram for gram. Something to think about next time you're coming down with a cold!

How Much Vitamin C Do I Need?

Adults need at least 40mg of vitamin C from food each day (a minimum of 10mg per day is required to prevent scurvy). One medium-sized red pepper contains around 130mg; a kiwi fruit and a 100g portion of steamed broccoli both contain around 60mg. While high-dose vitamin C may help to reduce the symptoms of some chronic health conditions, supplementation shouldn't exceed 1–2g per day without the advice of a health professional.

> **DID YOU KNOW?**
>
> Excessive levels of vitamin C supplements can irritate the digestive tract and may cause loose stools or diarrhoea.

Why Might I Be Low in Vitamin C?

- Your diet is low in fruit and vegetables
- You're a smoker: nicotine significantly depletes vitamin C in the body
- Regular consumption of alcohol reduces vitamin C levels
- You boil your vegetables: vitamin C is water soluble and around 45% of the vitamin C will leach out into the boiling water
- Certain medications may reduce levels of vitamin C
- Chronic stress and exposure to pollution both deplete vitamin C

3 Ways to Boost Your Vitamin C Levels

1. Favour vegetables over fruit when it comes to your 5-a-day. Gram for gram, you could easily double your dose of dietary vitamin C.
2. Steam your vegetables instead of boiling them, as this will help to conserve the nutrient content. Recent research also suggests that microwaving vegetables may help to reduce the possible loss of vitamin C because the exposure to heat is short-lived.
3. Limit your intake of alcohol and/or cigarettes to prevent the depletion of vitamin C in the body.

ZINC

You can find zinc in most foods, but there aren't many foods that are a standout source, which means that it's important to have a varied diet to ensure you're getting all the zinc you need on a daily basis. Top sources include oysters, lamb and pumpkin seeds, but you'll also find zinc in other shellfish, meat and poultry, nuts, seeds and vegetables in smaller quantities.

Why Do I Need Zinc?

Zinc is a mineral which is involved in almost all our vital functions, including reproduction and nerve function. A powerful antioxidant, it supports the immune system, promotes wound healing and helps to counteract the action of harmful free radicals.

How Does Zinc Help My Energy Levels?

Zinc is another key catalyst nutrient which activates the enzymes in the electron transport chain to help the body produce energy. Optimum zinc levels have been shown to improve athletic performance by increasing blood levels of testosterone, giving you a massive boost of Va Va Voom. A deficiency in zinc has been shown to increase insulin resistance, a condition where our cells no longer respond to insulin, the hormone required for the regulation of blood glucose levels. This can result in a state of constant fatigue.

DID YOU KNOW?

We need optimum levels of zinc in the body to maintain the correct levels of vitamin E in the blood and to support the absorption of vitamin A.

Typical Symptoms of Zinc Deficiency

- Poor sense of taste or smell
- Frequent colds or infections
- Fatigue
- Acne
- White marks on fingernails
- Low sperm count

- Loss of appetite
- Slow wound healing
- Loss of libido
- Delayed sexual maturation
- Low mood
- Thinning hair

How Much Zinc Do I Need?

Current advice is that adults need at least 7–10mg of zinc per day from food. A standard 100g portion of roasted or braised lamb contains about 5mg; 2 tablespoons (25g) of pumpkin seeds contain about 1.6mg. It's important not to exceed 25mg per day in supplement form without the advice of a health professional. Although zinc supports the immune system, daily doses of more than 1000mg in supplement form can depress the immune system and may lead to zinc toxicity.

DID YOU KNOW?

Unlike some vitamins and minerals, zinc has a relatively stable shelf life, which means levels are unlikely to be overly affected by lengthy storage of food. While plant sources such as lentils can lose up to 20% of zinc when cooked in water, meat sources generally retain most of their zinc during the cooking process.

Why Might I Be Low in Zinc?

- You're not eating a balanced diet
- Stress can deplete zinc levels in the body
- Regular alcohol consumption can block the absorption of zinc
- High levels of dietary grains: grains contain phytates which inhibit the absorption of zinc
- You're taking zinc and iron supplements at the same time and they are competing for absorption
- Zinc can be lost through excessive perspiration

- Inflammatory bowel conditions can affect absorption of zinc in the gut
- Chronic health conditions such as diabetes and kidney and liver disease are associated with low levels of zinc

3 Ways to Boost Your Zinc Levels

1. Snack on pumpkin seeds daily or add a tablespoon to your morning cereal, porridge or smoothie.
2. Make sure that you're not eating large amounts of wheat with every meal: wheat-based cereal for breakfast, sandwich for lunch and pasta for dinner, for example. Wheat is especially high in phytates which inhibit the absorption of zinc.
3. Avoid drinking alcohol every day and don't binge-drink when you do have alcohol, as this can dramatically reduce zinc levels in your blood.

COPPER

You may be surprised to learn that copper is an essential micronutrient if you're more familiar with it being used for the pipes in your plumbing. The best sources of copper tend to be plant foods, such as sesame seeds, cashews, mushrooms and green vegetables, although it can also been found in decent quantities in shellfish.

Why Do I Need Copper?

Although we only need tiny amounts of it, copper has a role in many essential systems. We need it to make collagen, a protein needed for healthy bones, skin and connective tissue. Copper supports the immune system and promotes wound healing. We also need copper to keep our nerves healthy.

How Does Copper Help My Energy Levels?

Copper has a dual role in supporting energy. Firstly, it acts as a catalyst in energy production, ensuring the process runs smoothly. Secondly, copper is required for the formation of haemoglobin, and is therefore essential for the transportation of oxygen to our cells. Low levels of copper can mimic symptoms of anaemia, leaving you feeling drained and weak.

DID YOU KNOW?

Copper deficiency impairs the immune system by disrupting the production of white blood cells and reducing the body's ability to fight infection.

Typical Symptoms of Copper Deficiency

- Anaemia
- Low bone density
- Stunted growth
- Fatigue
- Anxiety
- Poor memory
- Thinning hair or weak nails
- Skin sores
- Frequent colds or infections
- Joint or muscle pain

How Much Copper Do I Need?

We only need copper in very small amounts, roughly 1mg per day (from food). As copper is found in most foods in small quantities, eating a varied diet is likely to provide all the copper you need. 20 raw cashew nuts contain 0.4mg; 100g of prawns contain about 0.3mg and 2 large handfuls of baby spinach leaves contain about 0.15mg. Copper supplementation shouldn't exceed 1mg without the advice of a health professional. Copper works in very close synergy with other micronutrients, so it's probably best to take it as part of a multivitamin and mineral supplement, where you'd usually find it at 0.5mg or less, to ensure the correct balance. Excessive levels of copper in your system due to excess supplementation or exposure to environmental copper may result in copper toxicity which can have serious health implications.

DID YOU KNOW?

Copper and zinc work in opposition to each other, so that too much of one can lead to a deficiency of the other. If copper and zinc status is out of balance, this can lead to suboptimal thyroid function.

Why Might I Be Low in Copper?

- Excessive levels of zinc in the body
- You're not eating a balanced diet
- Long-term use of oral contraceptives may disrupt copper levels, by either increasing or decreasing it
- Chronic stress can deplete copper
- Poor absorption in the gut, due to suboptimal digestion

3 Ways to Boost Your Copper Levels

1. Avoid taking high doses of individual zinc supplements for a prolonged period of time.
2. Make sure you're eating a wholefoods diet with plenty of nuts, seeds and legumes, as these are naturally high in copper.
3. Opt for wholegrain foods such as wholemeal bread or brown rice; the refining process that removes the outer layer of the grain to create white flour or rice can halve the amount of copper.

CHOLINE

Choline is a water-soluble nutrient related to the B vitamin family and is a component of the molecule phosphatidylcholine, which is mostly found in foods that naturally contain some fat. Eggs are an excellent source of choline, but it can also be found in pulses, soya and cruciferous vegetables like broccoli or Brussels sprouts.

Why Do I Need Choline?

The body relies on choline for the communication process that sends signals from the brain to the rest of the central nervous system. It also helps with fat metabolism, regulating cholesterol and supporting heart function.

How Does Choline Help My Energy Levels?

Choline acts as a catalyst nutrient in the conversion of fuel into energy, helping to kick-start the citric acid cycle. Your internal engine may start to sputter if you're running low. It's also important for mental energy, promoting memory, concentration and focus through the synthesis of the acetylcholine neurotransmitter.

Typical Symptoms of Choline Deficiency

- Poor memory
- Loss of concentration
- High cholesterol
- Fatty liver
- Cardiovascular disease
- Difficulty digesting fatty foods
- Neurological disorders
- Low energy
- Aching muscles

DID YOU KNOW?

Excessive levels of choline can lead to a fishy body odour in some individuals who are unable to correctly break down some of its metabolites.

How Much Choline Do I Need?

Adults need about 550mg of dietary choline per day and it's found in many different sources. A single egg contains about 150mg of choline; a portion of broccoli contains about 60mg and a medium cod fillet contains about 90mg. There isn't currently a recommended daily amount for choline supplements but the standard dosage is 200–300mg and you should seek advice from your doctor before taking a higher dose.

DID YOU KNOW?

Choline and folate work in synergy and low levels of either can make it harder for the other to carry out all its essential functions.

Why Might I Be Low in Choline?

- Regular consumption of alcohol can deplete choline levels
- Poor nutrient absorption in the gut
- If you're reliant on plant sources of choline, remember that it's water soluble, so boiling vegetables will deplete choline levels
- Genetic factors may mean that some people use up more choline in the detoxification process
- Low levels of vitamin B or folate can lead to the body using choline as a substitute

3 Ways To Boost Your Choline Levels

1. Steaming instead of boiling vegetables will help to avoid the choline leaching out into the water.
2. Make sure you're not drinking alcohol every day as this will deplete choline levels.
3. Eat an egg 3–4 times per week.

IRON

Iron is found in two forms in food: iron which is attached to a haem protein and found in animal sources, such as meat, fish and eggs, and iron attached to a non-haem protein which is found in plant sources such as vegetables, pulses, nuts and seeds. Haem iron is absorbed far more effectively by the body than non-haem iron which may be something to consider if you follow a vegetarian diet.

Why Do I Need Iron?

Possibly the most important function of iron is its involvement in the production of haemoglobin and myoglobin, a form of haemoglobin found in the muscles, essential for the generation of energy for muscle contraction.

How Does Iron Help My Energy Levels?

If you're low in iron, you're likely to feel drained and weak because the oxygen that we need to make energy isn't reaching our body cells. Iron is an essential component of haemoglobin, the protein in our red blood cells that transports oxygen around the body, fuelling our brain, muscles, tissues and cells. Lack of oxygen would be a classic example of why our spark plugs might start to misfire.

Typical Symptoms of Iron Deficiency

- Anaemia
- Low energy and fatigue
- Headaches
- Pale skin
- Palpitations
- Sore tongue
- Loss of appetite
- Dizziness
- Brittle hair

DID YOU KNOW?

The absorption of plant (non-haem) sources of iron is far more easily influenced by other nutrients than animal (haem) sources. Vitamin C can help to increase the absorption of non-haem iron by up to 30%. Tea and coffee can significantly hinder the absorption of non-haem iron.

How Much Iron Do I Need?

Current advice is that men and non-menstruating women need around 8.7mg of iron from food each day. Menstruating women require nearly double that at 14.8mg. 100g of rump steak contains about 4mg of iron; an egg yolk contains about 0.5mg; 2 handfuls (about 50g) of raw baby spinach and a tablespoon of pumpkin seeds each contain about 1mg of iron. Iron supplements should only be taken if you've been diagnosed with anaemia. If you take a multivitamin and mineral supplement, it's best to choose a product that doesn't contain iron. Iron is stored in the body and a build-up of excessive iron in your tissues can lead to serious health issues. Supplement intake should not exceed 17mg per day without the advice of a health professional.

DID YOU KNOW?

Inorganic iron supplements, such as ferrous sulphate, are much harder for the body to absorb and may lead to nausea, cramping or constipation. Organic forms, such as ferrous fumarate or ferrous gluconate are easier for the body to deal with and more easily absorbed.

Why Might I Be Deficient in Iron?

- You follow a vegan diet: non-haem iron is less easily absorbed by the body
- Prolonged use of antacids and/or low levels of stomach acid can reduce iron absorption
- A deficiency of vitamins B6 or B12 can reduce iron absorption
- Blood loss due to heavy or prolonged menstruation or gastrointestinal bleeding
- Excessive consumption of tea or coffee
- High levels of dietary oxalates (found in spinach and rhubarb) or phytates (found in wheat bran and oats) can block iron absorption

3 Ways to Boost Your Iron Levels

1. Try opting for more unusual red meats than beef or lamb: venison contains twice as much iron per 100g as beef, and calf's liver contains four times as much.
2. Make a point of eating foods rich in vitamin C with plant sources of iron to maximise absorption e.g. roasted red peppers with tofu, or a green salad with lentil bake.
3. Don't take your iron supplements with tea or coffee – leave a gap of at least an hour before or after taking supplements to ensure optimum absorption.

AMINO ACIDS

There are 22 amino acids which are the building blocks of protein and they all have multiple roles in supporting the body. Of these, 9 are essential amino acids which need to be acquired through the diet. The body is able to synthesise the remaining amino acids that we need. Complete proteins contain all the essential amino acids and these can be found in one easy package in animal proteins, such as meat, fish or eggs. Plant proteins, such as pulses, nuts and seeds, tend to contain some but not all the essential amino acids which means that vegans may have to work harder to vary their diet in order to allow for the correct balance. Soya beans and quinoa are examples of plant foods which are complete proteins.

Why Do I Need Amino Acids?

Amino acids are vital for a whole range of metabolic functions: they combine to form proteins which we need for the growth, regeneration and repair of our body cells and tissues, as well as for hormone production. Some amino acids convert to neurotransmitters which act as chemical messengers throughout the body.

How Do Amino Acids Help My Energy Levels?

Certain amino acids play a particular role in supporting energy levels either directly as catalyst nutrients which fire up our internal engine or indirectly through their role in key systems of the body that impact our energy. The following amino acids could help increase your Va Va Voom:

Glutamine acts as fuel for the brain, supporting memory, focus and concentration. It also helps to build and maintain muscle strength and support gut function, enhancing optimal nutrient absorption.

Glycine improves glycogen storage, freeing up glucose for energy as our internal engine requires. It also helps to improve memory and mental performance.

Isoleucine is required for the formation of haemoglobin in our red blood cells which transports oxygen around the body, essential to fire up energy production in our cells. It also helps to regulate blood sugar levels. Isoleucine is one of 3 branched-chain amino acids that can enhance energy levels, increase endurance and improve athletic performance.

Leucine is another branched-chain amino acid that supports endurance and performance levels. It can also help to reduce high blood sugar.

Methionine plays a key part in the detoxification process, supporting digestion and protecting the liver from toxic overload which can be a drain on our energy levels – a bit like air draining from a tyre when it has a slow puncture.

Phenylalanine converts to tyrosine in the body; tyrosine is used to produce the neurotransmitter noradrenaline which promotes alertness and motivation and triggers the release of glucose from energy stores, taking you up a gear.

Tryptophan is converted in the body to the neurotransmitter serotonin, from which melatonin is synthesised. Melatonin regulates our sleep cycle and ensures that we wake refreshed and energised in the morning.

Tyrosine converts to noradrenaline, as we have seen above. It's also essential for optimum thyroid function. Low levels of tyrosine may result in a sluggish thyroid and low energy, because thyroid hormones regulate the way our body uses energy.

Valine is the third branched-chain amino acid, supporting muscle strength, repair and recovery and enhancing endurance and performance, so that your internal engine can power on throughout the day.

Typical Symptoms of Amino Acid Deficiency	
Glutamine	Poor exercise performance; digestive problems; impaired immune function; poor concentration and memory
Glycine	Increased inflammation; painful joint or muscles; poor digestion; poor sleep; low energy
Isoleucine	Headaches; dizziness; fatigue; lack of stamina; poor exercise performance, loss of muscle mass; craving for sugar or carbs
Leucine	Loss of muscle mass; dizziness and confusion; lack of stamina; cravings for sugar or carbs; poor exercise performance
Methionine	Fatty liver; low mood; lethargy; increased cholesterol; poor skin condition
Phenylalanine	Confusion; loss of focus; poor memory; low mood or depression; loss of energy and motivation
Tryptophan	Low mood or depression; anxiety; disrupted sleep; reduced ability to manage stress; carbohydrate craving
Tyrosine	Fatigue; weakness; poor thyroid function; aching muscles or joints; weight gain; sensitivity to the cold
Valine	Low energy; reduced muscle recovery; low muscle mass; poor exercise performance

DID YOU KNOW?

The body can't store amino acids for very long, so we need to be eating protein every day to maintain optimal levels for good health.

How Many Amino Acids Do I Need?

If you eat plenty of foods rich in complete protein, your body will do the rest by producing the remaining non-essential amino acids from the ones you've consumed in your diet. Amino acids are very powerful substances so beware of supplementing them individually in high doses without the advice of a health professional as this may disrupt neurotransmitter balance, which can be dangerous. If you're planning to use protein powders, perhaps to support your training regime, this may provide a more balanced approach but they're generally only required in cases of intense training, such as triathlon or marathon preparation. A standard hour at the gym can be supported adequately by a balanced diet.

Why Might I Be Low in Amino Acids?

- You're not eating enough complete protein and may be getting plenty of some amino acids but not others
- You're not eating protein every day
- Your body is unable to digest or absorb protein, which may be due to low levels of hydrochloric acid in the stomach
- Regular use of antacids may impair protein digestion, by reducing levels of stomach acid
- As we age, stomach acid levels drop which can make it harder to digest or absorb protein

DID YOU KNOW?

Chronic stress can reduce levels of hydrochloric acid in the stomach, making it very hard for the body to break down, digest and absorb complex proteins such as red meat. This can lead to bloating, flatulence and feeling over-full after even a small meal.

3 Ways to Boost Your Amino Acid Levels

1. Eat foods rich in complete protein, such as meat, fish, eggs, quinoa or soya beans.
2. Make sure that you eat some form of protein with every meal and snack.
3. Be careful not to overdo the antacids, unless they've been prescribed by your doctor.

ENGINE OIL

Every engine needs oil to lubricate the parts and make sure they work together well without overheating. The next series of Va Va Voom boosters may not be an intrinsic part of the energy-production process but they do act as your personal engine oil, making sure that everything is running smoothly, so you're able to produce energy easily and efficiently.

VITAMIN D

Vitamin D is so important to our health and wellbeing that it's actually produced by the body through exposure to sunlight and stored in our fat cells. There are limited food sources of Vitamin D but small amounts can be found in oily fish such as mackerel or salmon, dairy products and liver.

Why Do I Need Vitamin D?

Extensive research into vitamin D in recent years has revealed a role that extends far beyond the traditional view of supporting healthy bones and teeth. While this remains a key function, vitamin D also plays an essential part in the immune system, helping to protect the body from infection. Some studies suggest that vitamin D may help to reduce the risk of chronic conditions such as type 2 diabetes, cancer, cardiovascular disease, rheumatoid arthritis and multiple sclerosis. Low levels of vitamin D have also been associated with mental health conditions such as low mood, depression and anxiety.

How Does Vitamin D Help My Energy Levels?

While vitamin D doesn't play a direct role in energy production, if you regularly struggle with reduced physical and mental energy, poor concentration and low mood during the winter months, this may be due to a deficiency in vitamin D. Seasonal Affective Disorder which leads to lethargy may be caused or exacerbated by low levels of vitamin D. A lack of vitamin D may also contribute to insomnia. If you're concerned about your vitamin D levels, consult your doctor for a blood test.

DID YOU KNOW?

Adequate vitamin D levels are essential for supporting calcium absorption. A vitamin D deficiency may result in low levels of calcium which could have a serious impact on bone health.

Typical Symptoms of Vitamin D Deficiency

- Bone pain, back pain and muscle weakness
- Low mood or depression
- Lack of energy
- Insomnia
- Unexplained fatigue
- Rickets in children
- Increased susceptibility to colds and infections
- Seasonal Affective Disorder
- Poor wound healing

How Much Vitamin D Do I Need?

Vitamin D is measured in International Units (IU). IU is not a mathematical measure like micrograms, it's a variable measure that expresses how much active vitamin D is available in a supplement. Current advice in the UK is for children aged 1–4 to take a daily dose of 400IU all year round. Adults and children are advised to take 400IU of vitamin D daily throughout the winter, although adults are more likely to benefit from a higher daily dose of 1000–3000IU. If you spend little time outside or cover your skin when outside, a year-round dose is advisable. Excessive daily doses of vitamin D over a long period may result in toxicity so it's important to check in with your doctor from time to time for a blood test.

DID YOU KNOW?

Vitamin D is a fat-soluble vitamin that can be stored by the body, which means that you could take 10,000IU once a week instead of a smaller daily dose if that suits you better. Some studies have shown that this type of larger dose may improve vitamin D absorption.

Why Might I Be Deficient in Vitamin D?

- Lack of exposure to sunlight if you're housebound or tend to cover up when you go outside
- People with Asian, African or Afro-Caribbean heritage can be prone to vitamin D deficiency
- Consistent use of high-factor sunblock
- You eat a vegan diet and have limited exposure to sunshine
- Age: as we get older, our body becomes less efficient at converting and absorbing vitamin D from sunlight

3 Ways to Boost Your Vitamin D Levels

1. 10–15 minutes in the sunshine without sunscreen each day. Even just exposing your forearms could make a big difference. The timing will, of course, depend on the strength of the sun and how fair your skin is, so it's important to adjust this accordingly to protect your skin and avoid burning. Even exposure for a short time should allow enough sunshine to be absorbed to support your vitamin D levels. People with dark skin may need about 40 minutes, as darker skin contains pigments which protect against the sun.

2. Mackerel and salmon are among the best food sources of vitamin D. Eating this type of oily fish 3 times a week could help support vitamin D levels, especially if your exposure to sunlight is minimal.
3. Take a daily vitamin D supplement of 400IU for children and 1000–3000IU for adults.

EXERCISE

Statistics show that people in the developed world have a more sedentary lifestyle now than at any time in our history, which has major implications for our health and longevity. Exercise comes in many forms and doesn't have to involve a workout at the gym if that isn't your style. Cycling, swimming, dancing, yoga, racket sports, football, running and brisk walking are all effective forms of exercise which you can incorporate into your daily routine.

Why Do I Need to Exercise?

There are a number of short- and long-term benefits to regular exercise and physical activity. Not only does exercise increase our fitness, endurance, strength and flexibility, there is also overwhelming evidence that it reduces the risk of chronic disease such as cardiovascular disease, cancer and type 2 diabetes. Exercise helps with weight management and obesity and it protects against osteoporosis by improving bone density. Regular exercise also improves quality of sleep and is a key factor in supporting our mental health.

How Does Exercise Help My Energy Levels?

It may seem counterintuitive, but moderate exercise when you're feeling tired can help to perk you up considerably. We've seen in Chapter 1 the important role that oxygen plays in the energy-production process. Exercise improves our circulation, sending more oxygen around the body to our muscles, tissue and brain. Regular exercise helps to reduce the stress levels that can rob us of energy (see Chapter 4) and it also helps to support mental energy through the release of the neurochemicals serotonin and endorphins, which promote a sense of positivity, motivation and wellbeing. Even regular low impact exercise like walking can increase energy levels by up to 20% for someone with a sedentary lifestyle. Studies have also shown that on the days that people exercise they feel more alert and have improved mental performance.

Typical Signs That You're Not Getting Enough Exercise

- A feeling of sluggishness and lethargy
- Loss of motivation
- Weight gain
- Insomnia
- Poor bone density
- You get out of breath walking upstairs
- You lack strength in your arms or legs
- You have lower back pain
- You experience constipation
- You feel tired all the time

How Much Exercise Do I Need?

Adults should be getting at least 2.5 hours of moderate aerobic exercise (exercise that raises your heart rate and makes you breathe faster) every week, which can break down to 30 minutes a day or larger blocks of time across the week, depending on what suits you. It's important to ensure that you do some resistance work on top of this to build muscle strength. This might include working with weights or resistance bands or using your own body weight as resistance by doing push-ups, plank or yoga, for example. Strenuous activities such as digging the garden can also help to build muscle tone.

DID YOU KNOW?

While exercise can help to relieve stress levels,
excessive intense training may increase levels of
the stress hormone cortisol. If you have a very
stressful job, you may benefit from more gentle
forms of exercise such as yoga, which encourages
the practice of slow and steady breathing as you
work through the movements.

Why Might I Not Be Getting Enough Exercise?

- You have a busy or erratic schedule
- You have a sedentary lifestyle and avoid opportunities for
'free' exercise, such as taking the stairs instead of the lift
- You favour resistance work over aerobic work or vice versa
- You're paying for but not using your gym membership
- You use your gym membership but spend more time in
the sauna or the café area
- You exercise dutifully 3 hours a week but spend the rest of
the time sitting in front of a computer, TV or games console
- Procrastination

How Can I Increase My Exercise Levels?

Start by (honestly) auditing your current exercise output to assess
how much you're doing on a weekly basis and give some thought
to what actually motivates you, because this will help identify the
best approach for you.

For example, if you're consciously careful with money, you're
more likely to make sure you get your money's worth from a gym
membership by attending regularly. There's absolutely no point
belonging to a gym and paying a hefty monthly fee if you don't go.

A gym membership can be a simple and practical solution, as it's
a handy one-stop shop for machines, weights and classes. However,
if you're motivated by variety, you may want to think about mixing

it up across the week – perhaps include a trip to the pool, a drop-in Pilates, yoga or dance class, a climbing wall, cycling, a game of tennis or a round of golf.

You may find it easier to increase your activity levels by teaming up with an exercise buddy. This is a great way to ensure you stick to an exercise plan, because you won't want to let them down by not turning up and you can help motivate each other and share in the highs and lows of your performance.

Don't forget that there are lots of opportunities for 'free' exercise in our daily life – always walk up the stairs (even if it's only part of the way) instead of taking the lift; get off the train or bus a stop early and walk the rest of the way; put music on and dance while you're cooking dinner; do strenuous housework or gardening; walk to the local shops and carry your shopping home; get a dog or borrow a friend's dog to go walking!

DID YOU KNOW?

It's important to be active every day, rather than simply relying on your 3 hours at the gym, as a lack of general movement could cancel out any health benefits you're aiming for. Including 'free' exercise in your daily routine can make a big difference to your total activity levels.

3 Ways To Boost Your Exercise Levels

1. Find a form of exercise that you genuinely enjoy as this will make you far more likely to commit to it on a regular basis. Think outside the box and try something different like a salsa or ballroom dance class, kayaking or climbing if you think the gym isn't for you.
2. Make a point of maximising free exercise opportunities every day, such as taking the stairs or walking to the shops.
3. Planning is key: write your exercise times into your diary so that they're as important as any other appointment and they don't get dropped for something else.

MINDFULNESS

Mindfulness is all about being aware of where we are and what we're doing in a particular moment. Everyday mindfulness is not the same as meditation, which is when you actively set aside time to focus on something, although there is an overlap between the two. There are lots of different types of meditation, such as movement meditation, prayer meditation or music meditation. Mindfulness meditation is the active practice of being in the moment, paying attention to your breath and being aware of your thoughts, sensations or feelings but not allowing them to distract you from the movement of your breath.

How Does Mindfulness Affect Me?

Mindfulness has a positive impact in a number of areas and there is an increasing body of research into the health benefits, which include pain management, stress reduction and improved mental health. It can help to relieve symptoms of low mood, depression and anxiety. By regulating the body's stress response, mindfulness may also support a more robust immune function. Mindful eating can support weight loss and help to manage our appetite.

How Does Mindfulness Affect My Energy Levels?

Studies have shown that the practice of mindfulness meditation supports mental performance by improving concentration, focus and memory. By helping to reduce our stress levels, mindfulness enhances mood and motivation. It also increases our resilience, improving stamina and energy levels.

Typical Symptoms of a Lack of Mindfulness

- Poor concentration
- Inability to focus
- Poor judgement
- Weight gain
- Fatigue
- Mood swings

- Low mood
- Poor memory
- Being a poor listener

DID YOU KNOW?

Mindful eating, which involves taking the time to focus properly on a meal instead of eating at your desk or in front of the TV, supports weight loss by making you more aware of what and how much you're eating. Eating slowly and mindfully activates digestive enzymes and stimulates the satiety response that helps us know when we're full. The raisin mindfulness exercise, which is very easy to find online, is an excellent introduction to mindful eating.

How Often Should I Practise Mindfulness?

There are no specific guidelines on how often you need to practise mindfulness, but you'll find it easier to behave mindfully in your daily life if you regularly schedule in some time for a mindfulness exercise. If you're able to set aside 15 minutes a day to sit quietly, breathe and focus on the present, this could make a big difference to your energy and wellbeing.

How Can I Improve My Mindfulness?

The importance of mindfulness is increasingly recognised so it shouldn't be difficult to find a practice or activity that suits you. If you already practise yoga, or if you'd like to start, make sure you attend a class that includes some meditation or pranayama breathing exercises. There are many different approaches to yoga and every teacher has their own style, so it's worth trying a few classes until you find one that you like.

Take a long, hard look at your mobile phone or tablet and think about how much you allow it to become a distraction to the matter in hand. Try switching it off when you're spending quality time with friends or family or if you're working on an important project, so that you're giving all your attention to the moment. This can gradually help you to reduce separation anxiety or FOMO (fear of missing out) so that your wellbeing is less dependent on your digital devices and social media.

If a meditation or yoga class isn't for you, try using a mindfulness app instead. There are lots of free options available which provide short and simple guided mindfulness exercises. You can try it out privately at home and build up your confidence that way.

Even short bursts of mindfulness, such as stepping away from your desk, closing your eyes and taking 10 deep breaths can help to re-centre your thoughts, calm your nervous system and improve cognitive action.

DID YOU KNOW?

Many yoga classes practise a form of mindful meditation and breathing called pranayama at the beginning or end of a class. The focus on breathing correctly throughout a yoga sequence is a form of exercise meditation which can have a hugely calming effect.

What Might Be Stopping Me from Being Mindful?

- You're constantly checking your mobile phone or email
- You're too busy recording the moment for social media to actually live in the moment
- The combination of a busy work and family life leaves you short of 'me' time
- You think it sounds weird
- You find it too difficult
- Your mind keeps wandering
- You're too busy worrying about the past or the future

3 Ways to Improve Your Mindfulness

1. Take time out during a busy day to move away from your desk, close your eyes and take 10 deep breaths in and out.
2. Do a yoga class with pranayama at least once a week.
3. Download a mindfulness app and take 15 minutes a day to follow a guided mindfulness meditation.

Chapter 4
Va Va Voom Robbers

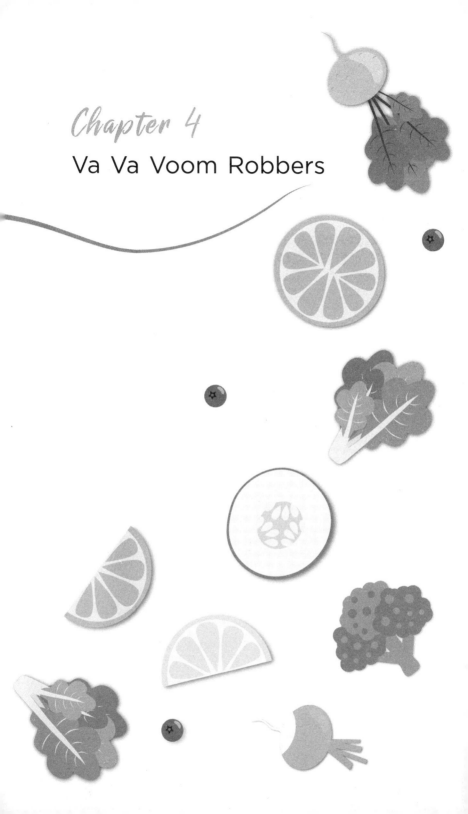

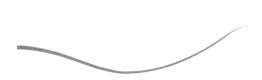

There are lots of different factors that can deplete energy in the body. Some are biochemical responses, such as inflammation or the insulin response to high blood sugar, and these are often a result of our chaotic 21st-century diet and lifestyle. Other factors relate to anti-nutrients that might block the absorption of Va Va Voom-boosting nutrients. Consuming too much of the wrong type of foods and drinks can also significantly disrupt the energy-production process so that our internal engine loses its Va Va Voom and begins to stall.

The Va Va Voom quiz may have identified certain Va Va Voom robbers that could be relevant to you, but it's worth checking out the others as well to see if you can establish a pattern that could be contributing to your lack of Va Va Voom.

CHRONIC INFLAMMATION

Inflammation is the first response of our immune system, an important line of defence to protect us against disease. It's activated by white blood cells which send chemicals to a site of injury or infection. This usually causes redness or swelling until the area is healed.

As a short-term response, inflammation can be a very effective part of the healing process. However, in some cases, inflammation occurs even when there are no foreign bodies to deal with. Over time, this chronic inflammation may lead to autoimmune conditions, where the body starts to attack its own tissues, or chronic health conditions such as cardiovascular disease or cancer. Inflammation can also cause common health niggles such as bloating or sinusitis.

How Does Chronic Inflammation Affect My Energy Levels?

Research has shown that fatigue is a common symptom of many inflammatory conditions and low-grade inflammation is increasingly recognised as an underlying factor in people who are TATT (tired all the time). People suffering from chronic fatigue syndrome often have high levels of inflammatory markers in the blood. Chronic inflammation can also result in a form of anaemia where the body doesn't have sufficient red blood cells to deliver oxygen around the body, leaving you feeling tired and weak.

Typical Symptoms of Chronic Inflammation

- Low mood or depression
- Feeling tired all the time
- A general sense of malaise
- Digestive cramping or bloating
- Painful muscles and joints
- Skin conditions such as eczema, dermatitis or acne
- High blood pressure
- Sinusitis or rhinitis
- Weight gain around the middle
- Allergies

Why Might I Have Chronic Inflammation?

- You have a bacterial infection in your stomach, small or large intestine
- You have an unidentified food allergy or intolerance
- Chronic stress can increase the production of inflammatory immune proteins called cytokines
- Your diet may feature too many foods that stimulate inflammation e.g. certain grains, red meat, dairy products, saturated fats and sugar
- You have an imbalance of gut bacteria, which can disrupt the immune cells in the gut wall, generating an inflammatory response
- Lifestyle factors such as insomnia, high levels of caffeine

or alcohol, dehydration and inactivity can all lead to inflammation

DID YOU KNOW?

Research has shown that following a Mediterranean diet can reduce the risk of contracting inflammatory conditions – but this doesn't mean more pasta and pizza! The Mediterranean Diet is rich in foods that have an anti-inflammatory effect on the body, such as fish, fresh fruit and vegetables, olive oil, nuts, seeds and herbs.

How Can I Manage My Inflammation Levels?

Diet is a key factor in inflammation: following a wholefoods diet rich in vegetables, fruit, pulses, fish, nuts and seeds will leave little room for pro-inflammatory foods such as certain grains, dairy, red meat and processed sugar. Consciously reducing levels of sugar, alcohol and caffeine will all help to relieve the inflammatory burden on the body. If you suspect a food sensitivity is at the root of your inflammation, it's important to identify and eliminate it (see page 99), as this could provide a very quick win. If you're planning to use an anti-inflammatory supplement such as fish oil, turmeric or ginger, always check with your doctor first to avoid any potential harmful interactions with medication.

Several other factors can also contribute to inflammation, so a multi-faceted approach may be more effective than simply focusing on one area. Addressing chronic stress by reviewing your working style, factoring in time for rest and relaxation and focusing on regular, gentle exercise can all help to relieve inflammation.

DID YOU KNOW?

The essential fatty acid omega 3 which is found in oily fish, nuts and seeds has a strong anti-inflammatory effect on the body. Too much of the essential fatty acid omega 6, however, can activate inflammatory pathways. Omega 6 is found in sunflower and corn oil, which feature in a lot of processed foods and ready meals.

3 Ways to Reduce Inflammation

1. Limit your intake of inflammatory foods, such as refined sugar, wheat, dairy products, red meat and alcohol.
2. Eat oily fish such as salmon, mackerel or sardines 3 times per week and add a tablespoon of ground flaxseed to your morning cereal.
3. If you're juggling a hectic work and family life, schedule in regular 'me' time when you can let your nervous system and stress levels calm down.

BLOOD SUGAR IMBALANCE

This is one of the most common lifestyle factors to affect energy levels. Every time our blood sugar drops, our energy levels drop with it. If you're prone to energy highs and lows throughout the day, you can be sure that blood sugar is the culprit. The infamous mid-afternoon energy slump is all about low blood glucose, usually as a result of a crash brought about by consuming too much refined sugar and carbohydrate, caffeine, alcohol or nicotine.

The body is programmed to keep levels of sugar in the blood within a very narrow limit, and this ensures sustained energy throughout the day. High levels of sugary food and refined carbohydrate cause a spike in blood sugar which generates the release of the hormone insulin in response. Insulin's job is to reduce sugar levels in the blood by storing it in the liver. Any excess sugar is stored in fat cells around the body.

The higher the spike in insulin, the lower the fall in blood sugar, which leads to a sugar 'crash'. This causes the stress hormones adrenaline and cortisol to be released. These hormones instruct the liver to release sugar stores into the blood as well as generating powerful cravings for a quick fix of sugar or carbs to redress the balance. This dual response will cause blood sugar to peak again, and so the vicious cycle of highs and lows continues throughout the day. Stimulants such as caffeine, alcohol and nicotine can also disrupt our blood sugar and insulin levels.

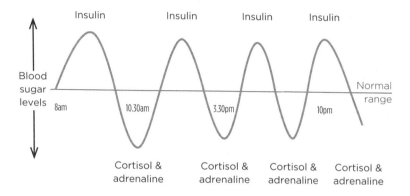

How Does a Blood Sugar Imbalance Affect My Energy Levels?

Sugar is a primary source of energy for the body so it's not surprising that if blood sugar levels are low you'll be feeling tired. Low blood sugar can also make you feel irritable, shaky, dizzy, anxious and can cause headaches. It will increase the levels of stress hormones in the body which won't help your energy levels if you're already experiencing chronic stress.

If your blood sugar constantly swings between high and low, the persistent battle of your hormones to keep things on the straight and narrow can be exhausting. A blood sugar imbalance will also affect the quality of your sleep. Going to bed with high blood sugar will activate insulin and your blood sugar will start to drop. As the stress hormones are released, you're likely to wake up in the middle of the night for no apparent reason or have a very restless sleep; by the time you wake up in the morning you'll feel tired and drained.

Typical Symptoms of a Blood Sugar Imbalance

- Energy peaks and troughs throughout the day
- Mid-afternoon munchies
- Cravings for sugary food or carbs
- Insomnia
- Headaches
- Dizziness
- A reliance on caffeine, sugar or alcohol to keep going
- Mood swings
- Poor concentration
- Irritability or anxiety
- Poor mental performance

Why Might I Have a Blood Sugar Imbalance?

- Your diet is high in refined sugar e.g. cakes, biscuits or chocolate
- You prefer refined carbohydrate such as white bread, white rice or white pasta to the wholegrain versions
- There's a lot of hidden sugar in your diet in the form of fruit juices or smoothies, sugary cereals or fruit yoghurts
- You drink too much tea, coffee or caffeinated fizzy drinks
- You regularly skip breakfast
- You don't eat enough protein
- Your diet is low in fibre
- You leave long gaps between meals

DID YOU KNOW?

Many apparently healthy foods such as breakfast cereals or fruit yoghurts contain surprisingly large amounts of sugar. 4g of sugar is the equivalent of a teaspoon, so make sure you check the label and do the maths if you want to regulate your sugar levels.

How Can I Balance My Blood Sugar?

The single best way to maintain a good blood sugar balance is to eat a combination of protein and fibre with every meal and snack. Good sources of protein include meat, fish, eggs, quinoa, pulses, nuts and seeds. Fibre is found in complex carbohydrate and good sources include vegetables, fruits with an edible skin, pulses and wholegrains like wholemeal bread or brown rice.

It's important to limit your intake of sugary foods, refined carbohydrate and stimulants such as caffeine, alcohol and nicotine, as all of these will stimulate the insulin response. Avoiding long gaps between meals is crucial. Even if you have the most balanced breakfast you can think of, if you leave it for 5 or 6 hours before you eat again, your blood sugar will start to drop. Everyone has a slightly different tolerance to blood sugar swings, but aim to eat a balanced meal or small snack roughly every 3–4 hours; adjust the timings to suit you and to maintain blood sugar levels and sustained energy.

Balance the proportion of your main meals carefully, so that protein-rich foods are about 25% of the meal; wholegrain starch (e.g. brown rice or wholemeal bread) is also 25% of the meal and vegetables make up 50% of the meal. If you're not eating starch at a meal, then increase the amount of vegetables to 75%.

> **DID YOU KNOW?**
>
> A standard 250ml glass of 'fresh' orange juice from a carton contains the equivalent of 5-6 teaspoons of sugar. One to watch if you're prone to knocking back the juice as one of your 5-a-day.

3 Ways to Balance Your Blood Sugar

1. Include protein in your morning cereal by adding a tablespoon of seeds, such as pumpkin or sunflower, or a handful of chopped nuts, such as walnuts or almonds.
2. Swap white starch for brown starch, so that you're eating

wholemeal bread, brown rice and wholegrain pasta or
noodles instead of the refined white versions.

3. Swap sugary snacks like biscuits or chocolate for some raw
   unsalted nuts with a piece of fruit or carrot sticks with 50g
   of houmous.

REFINED SUGAR

Refined sugar is natural raw sugar that has been broken down into
the form of pure white sugar, such as table sugar. It has a dual Va
Va Voom-robbing effect because it's highly inflammatory and it's a
key culprit in causing a blood sugar imbalance.

The obvious dietary sources of refined white sugar include sweets
and chocolate, cakes, biscuits, pastries and desserts, but it can also
be hidden in multiple other sources. Watch out for pasta sauces,
fruit yoghurts, jams, ready meals, soups and breakfast cereals. You
need to be careful of drinks as well. Lots of alcoholic drinks are
high in refined sugar, in particular beer, white wine, rosé and sparkling wine and liqueurs. Fruit juices and smoothies can be especially
high in sugar. Refined carbohydrate such as white bread, white
pasta and white rice is rapidly broken down into sugar by the body
and too much of any of these will lead to the same effects.

As we have seen in the blood sugar imbalance section above,
eating lots of refined sugar will trigger the insulin response, which
stores some sugar in the liver and encourages the body to store any
excess as fat. If you're constantly eating too much sugar your body
may become resistant to the action of insulin, making it impossible
to regulate blood sugar levels; this can lead to type 2 diabetes.

Refined sugar is highly inflammatory and is a key risk factor for
chronic disease. Excessive levels of refined sugar can disrupt the brain
and nervous system, causing a state of over-excitement followed by
feeling jittery or anxious as the sugar withdraws from your system.

How Does Refined Sugar Affect My Energy Levels?

If you're constantly reliant on sugary foods to keep you going, this
will lead to a series of blood sugar highs and lows throughout the

day, which will cause multiple dips in energy and may also disrupt your sleep.

If your diet is consistently high in sugar, you may be in a state of chronic low-grade inflammation due to the highly inflammatory nature of sugar. This can cause you to feel tired all the time.

Too much sugar can also affect your mental energy by disrupting neurotransmitter function, which can lead to poor memory and an inability to concentrate.

Typical Symptoms of Excess Sugar Consumption

- Weight gain
- Digestive discomfort
- Poor skin
- Dental Problems
- A sense of being tired all the time and needing a pick-me-up
- Joint pain
- Anxiety or nervousness
- Constant colds or infections
- High cholesterol
- High blood pressure
- Poor concentration and memory

Why Might I Have Too Much Refined Sugar in My Diet?

- You have a blood sugar imbalance so that your hormones are driving your food choices
- You have a sweet tooth
- You eat lots of foods that contain hidden sugars
- You eat a lot of white bread, white rice or white pasta
- You drink too much alcohol
- You add sugar to hot drinks
- You drink a lot of fruit juice or fizzy drinks
- You snack on cereal bars
- You eat a lot of dried fruit e.g. dates, dried apricots or raisins

DID YOU KNOW?

High levels of sugar in a man's diet may lead to erectile dysfunction because of its impact on blood vessels and circulation which can inhibit healthy blood flow.

How Can I Reduce the Refined Sugar in My Diet?

As we have seen in Chapter 3, sugar and carbohydrate are important sources of fuel which our body uses to produce energy. The trick is to achieve steady and sustained levels of energy over the course of the day rather than the highs and lows that come with using refined sugar as a quick energy fix.

Drawing our energy from complex carbohydrate such as vegetables, low-sugar fruits and wholegrain foods is a far more effective way of ensuring long-term Va Va Voom than relying on refined sugar. Combining protein with complex carbohydrate will help to buffer the impact of the sugars by slowing down their release into the bloodstream.

Limiting your intake of chocolate and sweets, desserts, biscuits, cakes and other baked goods can significantly reduce the levels of refined sugar in your diet. Check the labels on breakfast cereals, pasta sauces, ready meals and fruit yoghurts to assess the amount of sugar in the product. 4g of sugar is equivalent to a teaspoon, which will help you calculate how high in sugar your favourite food products really are.

Avoid fruit juices and fruit smoothies or opt for versions that contain a combination of fruit and vegetables to reduce the sugar load. Steer clear of sugary alcoholic drinks like white or rosé wines, sparkling wine and premium lagers.

DID YOU KNOW?

Honey, apple juice, dried fruit, fruit purée, fructose, dextrose, sucrose, maple syrup, corn syrup, dates and molasses are all just sugar under another name, so watch out for these when you're checking labels or trying new recipes.

3 Ways to Reduce Your Refined Sugar Intake

1. Eat wholegrain bread, brown rice and wholemeal pasta instead of the refined white versions.
2. Redefine your idea of a treat and have one no more than once a week, instead of every day (e.g. chocolate or any sugary option like sweets, biscuits, cakes etc).
3. Avoid sugary drinks: swap juices for cordials or mineral water and choose red wine or spirits such as gin or vodka instead of white wine, rosé or sparkling wine or beer.

WHEAT

While most grains are generally considered to encourage inflammation in the body, some grains are more problematic than others. Wheat has been selected as a potential Va Va Voom robber, partly because of the gluten content and partly because it tends to feature so strongly in our diet that it's likely to be a big culprit in increasing inflammation. Wheat is found in bread, breakfast cereal, pasta, noodles, couscous, cakes, biscuits, pastries and other baked goods. You'll also find wheat in beer, some vodkas and soy sauce.

Wheat contains a protein called gluten which becomes stronger and more elastic during the process of kneading bread or pastry. Anyone suffering from gluten intolerance will find wheat hard to digest and if you have coeliac disease, gluten will actively damage the gut and shouldn't be eaten in any form. Even if you don't have a diagnosed intolerance, gluten can be very hard on a sensitive digestion so if you're eating too much wheat, it's not uncommon to experience bloating, flatulence or inconsistent bowel movements.

Commercially produced products such as cereals, breads, pasta and baked goods are usually made with refined wheat flour. This is when the nutritious outer layer of the grain has been removed, and the fibre, vitamins and minerals along with it.

How Does Wheat Affect My Energy Levels?

Whether in wholegrain form or not, even a mild sensitivity to wheat could disrupt your digestive function, making it hard for the body to absorb key nutrients from your food, which will have a direct impact on the body's ability to produce energy.

Refined wheat products like white bread, white pasta and baked goods will be broken down into sugar very quickly by the body, due to the lack of fibre. If these feature regularly in your diet, you may experience the series of energy highs and lows that are characteristic of a blood sugar imbalance.

Typical Symptoms of Excess Wheat Consumption

- Bloating and flatulence
- Constipation or diarrhoea
- Weight gain
- Fatigue
- Brain fog
- Headaches
- Lethargy and drowsiness after eating

DID YOU KNOW?

Rye and spelt, which is an ancient form of wheat, both contain gluten but can be easier for some people to digest. This may be because the rye used in baking contains lower levels of gluten than wheat and the gluten in spelt is fragile, making it more vulnerable to the impact of heat. Either could be a more digestible option if you don't have coeliac disease but do have a mild gluten sensitivity.

Why Might I Have Too Much Wheat in My Diet?

- You typically eat wheat at every meal e.g. cereal for breakfast; a sandwich for lunch and pasta in the evening
- You drink large amounts of beer
- You regularly indulge in biscuits, cakes and pastries
- Your portions of bread, pasta or noodles are too big

How Can I Reduce the Wheat in My Diet?

Start by thinking more creatively about your meals and changing a few ingrained habits. Moving away from wheat- and bran-based cereals at breakfast time and opting for something made with oats, such as porridge, oat-based cereal, muesli or granola will remove both refined wheat and gluten. Swapping your lunchtime sandwich for a salad with either brown rice or quinoa as a base to add bulk could make a big difference to your energy levels in the afternoon. Cooking with potatoes or rice in the evening instead of being over-reliant on pasta will also help to reduce levels of wheat in your diet. Avoid snacking on biscuits, cakes and pastries and keep beer consumption to a minimum.

DID YOU KNOW?

The lengthy fermentation process involved in making sourdough bread helps to break down the gluten in the flour, which can make sourdough easier to digest than other types of bread.

3 Ways to Reduce Your Wheat Intake

1. Eat wheat at only one meal a day e.g. a wheat-based cereal OR a sandwich for lunch OR pasta for dinner.
2. Start snacking on fresh fruit with nuts or seeds or an oatcake with houmous, instead of biscuits, muffins and cakes when you need something to keep you going.
3. Swap wheat bread for 100% rye bread (check the label first, as lots of manufacturers use a blend of wheat and rye flour).

DAIRY

Dairy products are foods that contain or are made from cow's, sheep's or goat's milk. This includes butter, cheese, yoghurt, buttermilk, cream or ice cream. Baked goods such as cakes, biscuits and pastries usually contain dairy, as do most desserts and milk chocolate.

It's best not to be over-reliant on dairy as your main source of protein because it's a poorer source of protein than other animal foods such as eggs, meat and fish, which will keep you going for longer. Dairy is highly mucus-producing and sensitive individuals will experience nasal congestion and increased catarrh after eating too much dairy. Avoiding dairy if you have a cold or during the hay fever season, if you're a sufferer, can help to reduce congestion. While dairy is generally considered to be pro-inflammatory, natural yoghurt contains some beneficial bacteria due to the fermentation process. Eaten on a daily basis this can help to support a healthy digestive function, which is why natural yoghurt still features in the 10-day plan.

How Does Dairy Affect My Energy Levels?

Dairy foods, in particular milk and cheese, can stimulate an inflammatory response in some sensitive individuals. This may lead to bloating, constipation or loose stools, which will affect the absorption of key nutrients we need to produce energy. Intolerance to lactose (a milk sugar) or casein (a milk protein) will stimulate an immune response as the body seeks to protect us from a perceived threat. The low-grade inflammation that can develop as a result of an unidentified food sensitivity will deplete energy levels, leaving you feeling tired and low. Aged or very ripe cheese is high in histamine, an inflammatory chemical generated by the body during an allergic reaction. Some people are intolerant to the histamines which occur naturally in food and this can generate an immune reaction.

DID YOU KNOW?

While dairy is a quick and easy source of calcium, green vegetables, nuts and seeds contain almost double the amount per 100g and the soft bones in sardines make them one of the top calcium-rich foods.

Typical Symptoms of Excess Dairy Consumption

- Excess mucus production
- Catarrh
- Sinusitis
- Loose stools or constipation
- Eczema or dermatitis
- Bloating, wind or cramping
- Dark circles under the eyes
- Low energy

DID YOU KNOW?

Dairy is a common trigger for skin conditions like eczema or dermatitis, so you may benefit from reviewing your dairy intake if either of these are a problem for you.

Why Might I Have Too Much Dairy in My Diet?

- You add large amounts of milk to your morning cereal
- You drink 2 or 3 lattes every day
- You rehydrate with milk instead of water
- You eat cheese every day
- You use dairy as your main source of protein

How Can I Reduce the Dairy in My Diet?

There are lots of dairy-free milks such as soya, almond, oat, rice or coconut milk. You could try varying the milk you add to your morning cereal so that you're not over-reliant on cow's milk. If you're a regular at the coffee bar, steer clear of lattes, because these are mostly milk and will considerably add to your dairy tally.

If you're a vegetarian, broaden your protein sources to include more plant proteins, such as quinoa, pulses, nuts and seeds. This well help you avoid becoming over-reliant on dairy and ensure you're not tucking into cheese on a daily basis. Enjoy cheese a maximum of a couple of times a week.

3 Ways to Reduce Your Dairy Intake

1. Introduce dairy-free milk alternatives with your morning cereal or porridge so that you're not having large amounts of dairy in the morning.
2. Drink herbal tea or black coffee so that you're not topping up your dairy levels throughout the day.
3. Do your weekly shopping online. This will help you to stick to your shopping list and avoid being tempted by the offerings at the cheese counter.

EXCESSIVE CAFFEINE

Caffeine is a double-edged sword when it comes to your energy levels. There is no doubt that moderate amounts of caffeine provide a short-term burst of energy, which aids mental alertness. There is also a strong evidence base that caffeine can increase performance in endurance athletes.

However, there can be too much of a good thing and our over-reliance on caffeine to help us through our busy lives can have a strong negative effect on our energy levels. This is why it counts as a Va Va Voom robber. Caffeine is found in tea, coffee, caffeinated fizzy drinks, energy drinks and chocolate, as well as some painkillers and cold and flu medication.

Caffeine is a powerful natural stimulant and in excess it will disrupt the nervous system, causing restlessness, nervousness and anxiety. Too much caffeine can lead to high blood pressure and palpitations and make you feel jittery and over-excited. It can also upset the digestion.

How Does Excessive Caffeine Affect My Energy Levels?

The stimulating effect of caffeine can cause insomnia in sensitive individuals. It will also activate the insulin response, which can lead to a blood sugar crash and sap energy levels. High levels of caffeine also block the absorption of iron in the gut which we need for the production of haemoglobin and the transportation of oxygen to the cells for energy production. The addictive nature of caffeine can lead us to consume it throughout the day for a quick fix, which will increase the disruption to energy levels over time.

Typical Symptoms of Excessive Caffeine Consumption

- Insomnia or disturbed sleep
- Excitability
- Nervousness or anxiety
- Fatigue
- A feeling of being 'wired'

- Energy highs and lows
- Diarrhoea
- Acid reflux
- A racing heart
- Headaches

How Much Caffeine Should I Drink?

The recommended daily maximum for caffeine is 400mg which can easily be exceeded by having two large coffees from a coffee shop, depending on the dose they use. This information should be available from the barista or their website. Even 400mg may be too much for some people. Our ability to metabolise caffeine is highly individual so it's important to assess your own symptoms and have a lower dose if necessary, or stop consuming it earlier in the day if you know it affects your sleep. It's also important to remember that different sources of caffeine can easily add up over the day, so bear this in mind if you're having tea, coffee and caffeinated fizzy drinks, as well as chocolate.

DID YOU KNOW?

Green tea comes from the same plant as black tea and contains the same amount of caffeine. The longer you brew the tea, the stronger the caffeine content, so if you leave the bag in for 5 minutes rather than 1 or 2 minutes, it will roughly double the strength of the tea to about 75mg of caffeine.

Why Might My Caffeine Levels Be Excessive?

- The caffeine dose in your coffee is too strong
- You use energy drinks to keep you going
- You're addicted to chocolate
- You're drinking cups of tea throughout the day

- You're consuming multiple sources of caffeine without realising

DID YOU KNOW?

A 250ml can of a caffeinated energy drink contains around 80mg of caffeine and 7 teaspoons of sugar, a double whammy that will send your blood sugar soaring, setting you up for a major energy crash later in the day.

3 Ways to Reduce Your Caffeine Levels

1. Use less coffee if you're making it yourself or ask for one shot instead of two in a coffee bar.
2. Swap your caffeinated fizzy drinks for cordial and sparkling water if you need a bit of fizz.
3. Opt for caffeine-free tea or decaffeinated coffee from time to time.

ALCOHOL

While there's nothing wrong with enjoying the occasional tipple, there are increasingly alarming statistics about the excessive alcohol consumption across the general population. Historically men have consumed more alcohol than women but recent statistics have shown that women now drink the same amount as men. Hospital admissions related to alcohol consumption are increasing year on year.

Alcohol can affect our body in a number of ways. It's a powerful stimulant which disrupts the sympathetic nervous system, activating our 'fight or flight' response and increasing physiological stress on the body. It's important to remain within recommended limits because excess levels of alcohol increases our risk of chronic disease and can affect our mental health.

Much is made of the potential health benefits of some alcohol, in particular red wine, as it contains some protective antioxidants which may help to support heart health, reduce the risk of blood clots and regulate cholesterol levels. However, the evidence base is related to very moderate amounts, such as one small 125ml glass of wine per day or one 330ml bottle of lager. Any more than this will negate or even reverse any benefits you gained from the first drink.

How Does Alcohol Affect My Energy Levels?

You may feel that alcohol helps you get to sleep more quickly but its sedative effect disrupts your sleep cycle, limiting the amount of time in the deep sleep cycle and prolonging the restless REM (rapid eye movement) cycle which is when we dream. This can leave you feeling jaded and unrefreshed when you wake up in the morning.

Alcohol depletes our levels of the B vitamins that we need for the chain reaction of energy production and for the formation of red blood cells that carry oxygen around the body for our cells to produce energy.

Our blood sugar levels are affected by alcohol, partly because of the high levels of sugar in many alcoholic drinks and partly due to the stimulant nature of alcohol which will also activate the insulin response. This ultimately leads to a blood sugar crash, leaving you tired, irritable and dizzy. Excessive levels of alcohol will impair your liver function by keeping it very busy with the detoxification process. This can reduce its ability to metabolise energy which is one of its other important jobs.

Alcohol is a diuretic which leaves the body dehydrated and this reduces energy levels and both physical and mental performance.

Typical Symptoms of Excess Alcohol Consumption

- A hangover
- Poor-quality sleep
- Changes in behaviour or mood e.g. increased irritability, anger or forgetfulness
- Needing the toilet in the middle of the night
- Weight gain

- Dry eyes
- Low energy
- Dehydration
- Increased tolerance to alcohol
- Irregular heartbeat

DID YOU KNOW?

Giving up alcohol is a brilliant quick win if you're trying to lose your spare tyre. The high levels of sugar in many drinks, coupled with the disruption to your blood sugar levels and the activation of the stress response, all contribute to increased abdominal fat.

Why Might I Be Drinking Too Much Alcohol?

- Stress
- You don't realise how many units are in your favourite tipple
- You use alcohol to unwind
- You've got into the habit of drinking at home every night
- Peer pressure
- You binge-drink at weekends or when you go out

How Can I Regulate My Alcohol Consumption?

It's important to understand the concentration levels of the alcohol you're drinking. You may already know that the weekly recommended limit for men and women is 14 units, spread across the 7 days. But if you don't actually know what a unit is, this won't help you manage your alcohol consumption!

There are some very handy unit calculators online which you can use to precisely calculate the units in your favourite brands, but here's a rough guide in the meantime, based on average-strength products.

	Alcohol Units
Red Wine (175ml glass)	2.3
White Wine (175ml glass)	2.3
Rosé Wine (175ml glass)	2.3
Sparkling Wine (125ml glass)	1.7
Premium Lager (330ml bottle)	3
Bitter (1 pint)	2.3
Spirits e.g. gin, vodka, whisky (25ml single measure)	1
Fortified Wine e.g. port, sherry (per 50ml measure)	1

Drinking a glass of water in between each alcoholic drink can help to keep you hydrated and reduce some of the harmful effects of alcohol. Choosing smaller glasses of wine and having single instead of double measures of spirits will help to reduce your intake. A sparkling water with ice and lemon can easily pass for a gin and tonic or a vodka and soda if you're subject to peer pressure and want to slow things down on a night out.

DID YOU KNOW?

Going to the toilet in the middle of the night is probably nothing to do with your age, unless you're over 70. The body produces anti-diuretic hormone (ADH) at night time which concentrates our urine so that we don't produce as much and don't need to use the toilet. Production of ADH is reduced by alcohol, so we produce more urine after we've been drinking.

3 Ways to Reduce Your Alcohol Intake

1. Have at least 3 consecutive alcohol-free days each week to give your liver a break.
2. Ordering wine by the glass instead of a bottle when you're

out and about will help you keep track of what you're drinking. Avoid large 250ml glasses of wine as just 3 of these add up to a bottle.

3. Offer to be the designated driver on a night out – it's a very handy way of avoiding peer pressure!

DEHYDRATION

Over 60% of our body is made up of water and it's vitally important for the healthy functioning of all our body cells, tissues and organs. Dehydration occurs when the body loses more fluid than it takes in, which affects the optimal functioning of all key systems.

Every body cell needs water to function properly, and headaches and thirst are classic early warning signs that you're dehydrated. Deyhdration can affect you in lots of different ways, including constipation, dry skin and kidney infections.

How Does Dehydration Affect My Energy Levels?

Water is essential for our circulatory system, ensuring effective delivery of nutrients and oxygen around the body to support energy metabolism. Just 2% dehydration can significantly decrease our physical performance by affecting speed, strength and stamina. If our brain is starved of water, our mental energy is severely affected, leading to poor concentration, lack of creativity and confusion.

Typical Symptoms of Dehydration

- Thirst
- Fatigue
- Constipation
- Dry, rough or flaky skin
- Dry eyes
- Headaches
- Muscle or joint pain
- Dizziness or light-headedness
- Confusion
- Palpitations
- Poor mental and physical performance

DID YOU KNOW?

Dehydration often masquerades as hunger, so try drinking a glass of water next time you feel peckish as it may be all you need.

How Much Water Do I Need?

The amount of water you need varies according to your age, build, level of physical activity and the temperature of your environment, which means that it will be different for each person. Your intake of water should be enough to prevent you getting thirsty over long periods and to ensure that your urine is a pale straw colour.

Why Might I Be Dehydrated?

- Your fluid intake is low
- You've experienced diarrhoea or vomiting
- Excessive sweating can cause dehydration
- You're working or living in a hot environment
- You have heat stroke
- You've undertaken intense physical activity
- You've drunk too much alcohol
- Your blood glucose levels are high

How Can I Avoid Dehydration?

Drinking plenty of water throughout the day is the best way to ensure you're having all the fluid you need. If you don't like water or find it boring, try adding concentrated cordials or squash. Using sparkling mineral water can make it seem more exciting, although avoid if you have a sensitive digestion as it may increase bloating or wind. Herbal or fruit teas are a good way to boost your hydration. It's also worth noting that fruit and vegetables are full of water so eating plenty of these can provide an extra hydration boost. Tea, coffee and caffeinated soft drinks have a mild diuretic effect, so drinking these may result in a small net loss of fluid.

DID YOU KNOW?

Sparkling mineral water and soda water aren't the same thing. Sparkling mineral water is naturally carbonated and is bottled directly from the spring so the bubbles are completely natural, unless it's specifically labelled as carbonated mineral water. Soda water is plain water which has been artificially carbonated and may have additives, so it's a less natural option.

3 Ways to Avoid Dehydration

1. Keep an eye on the colour of your urine and assess the average over a 24-hour period as this will help you track your hydration patterns. Urine should be a pale straw colour – if it's darker, then you may be dehydrated and if it's completely clear, then you may be over-hydrated.
2. Eat 5–7 portions of fruit and vegetables every day.
3. Invest in a water app: if you tend to forget to drink, there are lots of handy apps that can help you keep on track via your smartphone.

FOOD SENSITIVITIES

Sensitivity to a particular compound in a food or drink can cause a series of inflammatory responses, as the body identifies a possible threat and generates a number of unpleasant symptoms.

Food sensitivities can feature as an allergic reaction triggered by the IgE antibody or as an intolerance triggered by the IgG antibody. An allergic reaction is an acute response with immediate symptoms such as vomiting, hives, skin rashes, swollen lips, wheezing or sneezing. A severe allergic reaction may lead to anaphylactic shock which can be life-threatening and which needs urgent medical treatment. The symptoms of an intolerance reaction may take up to 72 hours to show and they tend to develop into chronic health issues, such as digestive problems, eczema or other skin conditions, migraines, joint pain, difficulty losing weight and low mood.

How Does a Food Sensitivity Affect My Energy Levels?

If you've been struggling with an unidentified food sensitivity for a long time, this will result in a state of chronic low-grade inflammation in the body, which will have a direct impact on your energy levels. A food sensitivity commonly disrupts digestive function, causing symptoms such as bloating, flatulence, loose stools or constipation – all of which will impair the body's ability to absorb the nutrients we need to produce energy.

DID YOU KNOW?

Gluten intolerance is a symptom of coeliac disease but it's not the same thing as coeliac disease. It's perfectly possible to be intolerant to gluten and not have coeliac disease. However, it's impossible to have coeliac disease and not have gluten intolerance.

Typical Symptoms of a Food Sensitivity

- Bloating and wind
- Diarrhoea or constipation
- Vomiting
- Respiratory problems
- Swelling of the mouth, lips or tongue
- Skin conditions such as hives, eczema or dermatitis
- Fatigue
- Low mood
- Joint or muscle pain
- Headaches or migraine
- Extreme tiredness or lethargy soon after eating

- Excess mucus production
- Brain fog
- Post-nasal drip
- Itchy skin
- Regular colds and infections
- Unexplained weight loss or weight gain

What Might Be Causing a Food Sensitivity?

- You may have coeliac disease, an autoimmune condition which is characterised by an intolerance to gluten
- You may be deficient in the enzymes which are needed to digest lactose, a milk sugar
- You may be reacting to foods which are high in histamine
- You may have a chemical sensitivity to certain food additives or preservatives
- An imbalance in your gut bacteria is a common cause of delayed-onset food intolerance
- Stress or trauma can trigger food sensitivities
- Some people react badly to the nightshade family of vegetables and experience severe joint pain when they eat potatoes, peppers, tomatoes and aubergines

DID YOU KNOW?

Instead of being sensitive to one specific food, some people are sensitive to foods that contain high levels of histamine. Histamine is released as part of the inflammatory immune response in reaction to a potential harmful foreign substance in our body. Foods that naturally contain histamine include cured meats such as salami and bacon, smoked fish, fermented foods like sauerkraut or vinegar, beer and wine and some nuts such as walnuts and peanuts.

How Can I Find Out If I Have a Food Sensitivity?

Start by discussing it with your doctor who will be able to help with blood tests, skin prick tests or patch tests to identify a possible allergy and to rule out coeliac disease.

Keeping a food and symptom diary is a good next step if you suspect that you have an intolerance rather than an allergy, as you may be able to link a flare-up of your symptoms with a specific food or food group.

If you already have a suspicion about a food that may be a problem for you, then the best way to approach it is to do an elimination diet of that food for 3–4 weeks and observe your symptoms. It's important to plan your elimination carefully, especially if it's a major food group like dairy or wheat. Firstly, these foods feature in the ingredients of lots of different products, so it's worth doing a bit of research initially to identify common foods that contain your particular trigger. Secondly, you need to plan your diet carefully to make sure that it's still balanced and that you're eating plenty of other sources of key nutrients (such as calcium if you're eliminating dairy, for example).

A successful elimination diet relies on consistency. It's important to remove the food completely from your diet to achieve a meaningful result and you may benefit from working with a nutrition professional to help you get it right.

The reintroduction phase is the most important part of the elimination diet as this will help you identify whether a specific food is a potential trigger for you. It's important to start slowly, so you can easily observe any small changes. Have a portion of the food and leave it for several days because it can take up to 72 hours for symptoms to show. If you don't have any adverse symptoms, have another portion about 5 days later and leave it again for a few days. Over a period of weeks, build up your intake of the food, observing the symptoms along the way and stopping if you experience any unpleasant reactions. This will help you identify your own personal limits with the potential trigger food.

If this seems too much like hard work or you're struggling to identify the specific trigger, you may benefit from an IgG food intolerance test which is a finger prick test you can do privately.

3 Ways to Identify a Potential Food Sensitivity

1. Keep a food and symptom diary to help you identify potential triggers.
2. Try eliminating the trigger food <u>completely</u> for 3–4 weeks and observe your symptoms. It's best to do this one food at a time if you suspect you might be intolerant to more than one. Then reintroduce the food gradually (see previous page).
3. Consult your doctor or another health professional for advice about food allergy or intolerance testing.

SLUGGISH LIVER

'Sluggish liver' is a rather loose term to indicate that the liver isn't working as well as it might. It doesn't mean that you have liver disease, although it's always best to consult your doctor if you have any concerns. In the Va Va Voom-robber context it simply means that the liver might be struggling to keep up with things.

Although we tend to think of the liver as the 'detox' organ, it actually has more than 500 vital functions. In the same way that we might get bogged down with one project to the detriment of other projects at work, if the liver gets too busy clearing out toxins, it may struggle to keep up with its other responsibilities. Caffeine, alcohol and nicotine are examples of common consumable toxins. The liver is also required to process medication and old hormones and deal with environmental toxins, such as pollution or pesticides.

The liver deals with these toxins by chemically changing them and breaking them down. If your liver is over-worked, it may lead to a build-up of toxins and there may be disruption to some of its other key functions, such as hormone production, fighting infection and metabolising fat.

How Does a Sluggish Liver Affect My Energy Levels?

One of the key functions of the liver is the conversion of carbohydrate, fat and protein into energy. The liver is also critical in the control of the concentration of glucose (sugar) in our bloodstream, storing or manufacturing glucose as the body requires, which is a key factor in maintaining blood sugar balance and sustained energy levels. The liver is a storage site for energy-boosting iron and vitamin B12, which we need for the production and action of red blood cells.

Regular exposure to toxins in our diet, lifestyle and environment can keep our liver very busy, diverting its attention to the detoxification process and this can often cause constant low-level fatigue or sluggishness. In parallel to this, a build-up of toxins can disrupt the function of our mitochondria, where our energy production occurs.

Typical Symptoms of a Sluggish Liver

- Fatigue or lethargy
- Poor digestion
- Difficulty digesting fatty foods
- Headaches or nausea
- Excessive sweating
- Bad breath
- Eczema, dermatitis or psoriasis
- Weight gain
- Abdominal pain
- Acne, spots or skin rashes
- Aching muscles and joints
- Chronic fatigue syndrome
- Brain fog
- Low mood

What Might Be Causing a Sluggish Liver?

- Excessive alcohol consumption
- Exposure to heavy metals and pollutants such as mercury, lead, petrochemicals or pesticides
- Exposure to environmental toxins, moulds or fungus
- Food sensitivities
- High levels of sugar or processed food in your diet
- A lack of fruit and vegetables in your diet
- Excessive caffeine consumption
- Regular use of painkillers or other medication
- Smoking or recreational drug use

DID YOU KNOW?

Too much fructose, which is a form of fruit sugar,
isn't stored in our fat cells in the same way as excess
glucose. In fact, it's stored in the liver and high levels
of fructose in the diet can lead to non-alcoholic fatty
liver disease. This is mainly a concern if you consume
a large number of soft drinks or confectionery that
contain an extremely concentrated form of fructose
called high fructose corn syrup.

How Can I Avoid a Sluggish Liver?

Adjusting your diet and lifestyle can make a big difference to the
efficiency of your liver. Start by taking a hard look at how much alcohol
you drink. Whether you drink what you consider to be a moderate
amount every day or whether you save it up for a binge on a big night
out, your alcohol consumption might be making your liver work harder
than you imagine. Make sure that you're not exceeding the recommended weekly limit of 14 units (see pages 95–6). Avoiding alcohol
for at least 3 consecutive days each week will give your liver precious
time to focus on some of its other many jobs.

The liver relies on certain vitamins, minerals and plant compounds
to support the chain reaction of detoxification, so eating plenty of
vegetables, fruit and wholegrains can help to keep these processes
running smoothly, while keeping toxin levels to a minimum.
Cruciferous vegetables like broccoli and cabbage are particularly
supportive to the liver and vitamin C is a major player in detoxification as it directly supports the pathway which is responsible for
about 60% of the detoxification in the liver, breaking down alcohol,
nicotine, paracetamol, antibiotics and heavy metals. Where possible,
opting for organic fruit and vegetables will help to reduce the
exposure to pesticides and fungicides.

Limiting your intake of refined sugar will avoid putting too much
pressure on the liver to store the excess and convert it into glycogen.

It's also advisable to avoid processed foods and fast food as these are usually high in artificial additives and preservatives and can put an extra strain on the liver.

DID YOU KNOW?

Regular exercise can make a big difference to your liver function because it improves circulation of the blood and promotes the cleansing action of the liver. Studies have shown that it can help to reduce levels of inflammation in non-alcoholic fatty liver disease.

3 Ways to Avoid a Sluggish Liver

1. Make sure you have several consecutive alcohol-free days each week and don't exceed the weekly recommended level of 14 units of alcohol on the other days.
2. Eat a portion of cruciferous vegetables such as broccoli, cabbage, Brussels sprouts, cauliflower or pak choi 3 times per week.
3. Eat a wholefoods diet where foods are easily recognisable in their original form e.g. a fresh chicken breast rather than eating chicken as part of a processed or fast food meal. This will help to limit your exposure to artificial additives and preservatives.

POOR NUTRIENT ABSORPTION

The food we eat is broken down at different stages of the digestive system and absorbed into the bloodstream in the intestines. Digestion actually starts in the mouth with the release of digestive enzymes as we chew our food; it continues on through the stomach and into the small intestine, where most of the absorption takes place, and then into the large intestine or colon.

Poor nutrient absorption is mainly a result of a fault in one or more of these key sites of digestion, and it can lead to a number of unpleasant symptoms in the stomach and small and large intestines. All our body systems including the immune system, the cardiovascular system, the reproductive system and the nervous system, rely on optimal levels of certain nutrients, so poor nutrient absorption can disrupt any of these. This can lead to a wide range of symptoms relevant to each specific system.

How Does Poor Nutrient Absorption Affect My Energy Levels?

If your digestion isn't working properly then you won't be able to correctly absorb all the Va Va Voom boosters (see Chapter 3). These include key macronutrients, such as carbohydrate or fat, which provide the fuel we need to make energy, and the essential vitamins and minerals that act as important catalysts in the energy-production process. If nutrient absorption is a problem for you, you'll feel weak and lethargic.

Typical Symptoms of Poor Nutrient Absorption

- Low energy or fatigue
- Bloating and flatulence
- Constipation or diarrhoea
- Poor immune function
- Weight loss
- Slow growth
- Anaemia
- Thinning hair or brittle nails
- Poor skin
- Insomnia
- Loss of muscle tone
- Aching joints or muscles
- Low mood or depression
- Anxiety
- Poor concentration and memory

DID YOU KNOW?

A good way to check your gut transit time, which is the speed that food moves through your digestive system, is to eat a portion of beetroot and keep an eye on your stools over the next day or two; look out for a pinkish stool which has been stained by the beetroot. Food usually takes 12–24 hours to pass through the system, depending on how hard it is for the body to digest. Anything less than 12 hours may indicate poor absorption if food is passing too rapidly through the system.

What Might Be Causing Poor Nutrient Absorption?

- Inflammatory bowel disease, such as Crohn's disease or ulcerative colitis
- Coeliac disease
- A lack of beneficial bacteria in the gut
- Irritable bowel syndrome (IBS), a condition which can cause bloating, flatulence, constipation or diarrhoea
- Low levels of hydrochloric acid in the stomach, which prevents the absorption of iron and vitamin B12
- The body isn't producing enough digestive enzymes
- High levels of stress, which depletes B vitamins and magnesium
- Alcohol inhibits the absorption of B vitamins and vitamin C
- Tea and coffee reduces iron absorption
- A food allergy or intolerance
- A lack of fibre in the diet
- A high-sugar diet
- Diarrhoea
- Not chewing food properly
- Bacterial infection

DID YOU KNOW?

High doses of antibiotics can deplete the beneficial bacteria in the gut which may lead to problems with digestion and absorption. Eating fermented foods such as sauerkraut, tempeh and kimchi, or taking a good-quality probiotic capsule, will help to replenish your beneficial bacteria. The small amounts of beneficial bacteria in a daily dose of natural yoghurt act as a good maintenance dose.

3 Ways to Improve Your Nutrient Absorption

1. Support your digestion by eating foods that are rich in fibre, such as vegetables and wholegrains.
2. Improve levels of beneficial bacteria by eating fermented foods such as sauerkraut, kimchi and natural yoghurt on a regular basis.
3. Limit your intake of alcohol, caffeine and sugar because all of these impair nutrient absorption.

CHRONIC STRESS

Our stress response is designed to be a short-lived reaction of alarm in the face of a physical danger. However, the constant pressure of our 21st-century lives keeps many of us in a prolonged state of chronic stress. Our 'stress hormone' cortisol can remain constantly elevated as our sympathetic nervous system becomes dominant, so that we remain on red alert, suppressing our parasympathetic response which encourages a state of calm and relaxation.

Although we often think of stress as a negative state, it actually plays an important part in protecting us, by releasing stress hormones such as cortisol and adrenaline which act as shock absorbers to help us cope with difficult situations. Our stress hormones have a primitive reaction which is designed to protect us from imminent physical danger, such as a predator. A number of biological changes take place as part of the stress response and these can become problematic if we remain in a state of constant stress. Blood will be diverted to the muscles to make us faster and stronger, and it is diverted away from systems that are perceived as non-essential in the face of immediate danger, such as the digestive, reproductive or immune systems.

Therefore, chronic stress can disrupt the function of these important systems, leading to symptoms of IBS or frequent colds or infections, and it can even affect fertility. High levels of cortisol will also constrict the blood vessels and speed up your heart rate which may lead to long-term health issues such as high blood pressure.

How Does Chronic Stress Affect My Energy Levels?

If we're exposed to stress over a long period of time, the high levels of cortisol will encourage the body to conserve its resources for the moment of attack by increasing abdominal fat, rather than processing sugar as energy. Our cortisol levels are designed to fluctuate during the day: they will start to rise at about 5am so that we have the energy and impetus to spring out of bed when we wake up; they fall gradually throughout the day with a steep decline at around 10pm, so that our body relaxes and is ready for sleep. Chronic stress can subvert this rhythm, so that we get a 'second wind' of energy in the evening, which can make it hard to switch off and get to sleep and therefore we feel tired and drained in the morning. Over time, chronic stress can lead to a state of severe fatigue or burnout.

Typical Symptoms of Chronic Stress

- Difficulty switching off
- Increased irritability
- Exhaustion
- Abdominal weight gain
- Loss of libido
- Sugar or salt cravings
- Frequent colds or infections
- Loss of motivation
- Poor concentration and memory

- A sense of being overwhelmed
- Dizziness when standing up
- Sleeping too much or too little

What Might Be Causing Chronic Stress?

- Poor work–life balance
- Major life changes
- Lack of rest and recuperation
- Financial problems
- Relationship difficulties
- Family health issues
- Bereavement
- Caring responsibilities
- Trauma
- Illness or injury
- Divorce

DID YOU KNOW?

The practice of mindfulness helps to reconnect us with our body and encourages us to be in the moment. Research has shown that this can have significant benefits in psychological health and stress reduction.

How Can I Manage My Stress?

While the logical thing might be to remove the source of your stress, this isn't always possible or practical. However, you can put in place some diet and lifestyle strategies that will help to support the body's response to stress and provide you with some coping mechanisms. One significant change you can make is to keep your blood sugar balanced (see page 78). Every time your blood sugar drops, your body will release cortisol and adrenaline to help redress the balance. Your lifestyle is probably stressful enough as it is, without generating more stress hormones!

Magnesium, B vitamins and vitamin C all support the action of your adrenal glands, which act as your internal shock absorbers and regulate the production of stress hormones, so eating plenty of wholegrains and leafy green vegetables can make a big difference to how well you manage your stress.

Limiting your reliance on food and drink that stimulate the stress response is important. Reducing your intake of caffeine, alcohol and sugar will be a big help.

Lifestyle is also a huge factor in managing stress levels. Try to factor in 'me' time on a regular basis; take control of your schedule and allow yourself to say 'no' from time to time, so that you get some downtime and headspace; take a short break away from your desk to give yourself a breather; focus on activities you find relaxing, like massage, reading, saunas or walking in nature; take regular exercise and add a yoga class into the mix; try a meditation class or download an app that you can follow.

DID YOU KNOW?

Closing your eyes, standing up and taking 10 deep breaths in and out can help to reduce blood pressure, calm down your stress response and improve the flow of energy to the body and brain.

3 Ways to Reduce Your Stress Levels

1. Try an Epsom salts (magnesium sulphate) bath after a stressful day. Add 2–3 handfuls to the bath with no other bath product. The magnesium will be absorbed through the skin, calming the nervous system and relieving muscle tension.
2. Follow a blood sugar-balancing diet by eating a combination of protein and fibre with every meal and snack (see page 78).
3. Download a meditation or mindfulness app or sign up for a short course if this would suit you better.

INSOMNIA

Most of us are affected by insomnia at some point in our lives. If you regularly struggle to get to sleep, stay asleep, have disturbed or poor-quality sleep then you've been struck by insomnia.

Research has shown that sleep is about far more than just rest and if you struggle with insomnia you'll be missing out on some crucial support. While we're asleep, our body is undertaking an intensive process of restoration to keep us at peak health. All the cells in our body repair, recover and regenerate overnight which makes quality sleep essential for anyone recovering from illness or injury. Our immune system is hard at work producing protective antibodies to fight off infections.

The brain undertakes a self-cleaning process during sleep, removing potentially harmful proteins that build up during the day and which can lead to chronic mental health conditions such as dementia or Alzheimer's. During sleep we convert short-term memory to long-term memory which helps us retain information that we've learned during the day. Creative thought processes can also be helped during sleep because the brain has time to make neural connections, helping you to solve problems or find solutions which might have challenged you the day before.

How Does Insomnia Affect My Energy Levels?

Insomnia will obviously affect physical energy; if you're short of sleep you'll find it hard to get started in the morning and will feel tired during the day. This will be exacerbated if your insomnia lasts over several days. A lack of sleep will also affect your mental energy, leading to poor concentration, judgement and memory. You're more likely to make impulsive decisions and you will lack the energy and resources to think creatively.

Typical Symptoms of Insomnia

- Tiredness and low energy
- Poor concentration
- Irritability
- Increased intolerance towards people or situations

- Poor wound healing
- Constant colds and infections
- Weight gain
- Lack of memory
- Difficulty getting to or staying asleep
- Difficulty getting back to sleep if you wake up in the night
- Feeling unrefreshed when you wake up in the morning
- Depression or anxiety

Why Might I Have Insomnia?

- Stress
- Irregular sleep patterns such as frequent long-haul travel or shift work
- Having a heavy meal or eating too late at night
- You have a poor sleep environment
- You have a blood sugar imbalance
- You have a mental health disorder such as anxiety or depression
- You have an inactive lifestyle
- Your sleep patterns are disrupted by alcohol, nicotine or caffeine
- You're going through the menopause
- You're getting older: sleep patterns can change after the age of 60

DID YOU KNOW?

Magnesium has a calming effect on the body which is very effective for anyone struggling to get to sleep. An Epsom salts (magnesium sulphate) bath before bed relaxes the muscles and the nervous system, setting you up for a good night's sleep.

How Can I Manage My Insomnia?

Start by taking a close look at what you're eating and drinking in the evening. High levels of sugary foods, refined carbohydrate and alcohol will all send your blood sugar soaring just before bed. You might drop off to sleep easily enough but in the background insulin is getting to work, setting you up for a blood sugar crash that will wake you up 2 or 3 hours later.

Audit your caffeine levels and experiment with different cut-off times during the day to see if this improves your sleep. Remember that caffeine is found in colas, energy drinks, green and black tea as well as coffee and chocolate, so make sure you're not consuming it without realising.

Foods like milk, turkey or oats all contain the amino acid L-tryptophan which can help to improve sleep. The body converts tryptophan to serotonin and serotonin to melatonin, which is the hormone that regulates our sleep cycle. However, the amino acid L-tyramine generates the stimulating neurotransmitter noradrenaline, which promotes alertness, arousal and motivation. Foods rich in tyramine include processed meat such as bacon and salami and aged cheese and these are best avoided late at night.

If your bedroom is too hot, too cold, too noisy or too light, or if your bed is uncomfortable, this can affect the quality of your sleep. Consider ear plugs, eye masks, black-out blinds and layers instead of one thick duvet or quilt.

Ban digital devices from the bedroom! Tablets, smartphones and laptops all emit a blue light that disrupt the hormone melatonin that governs our sleep cycles. They also have a highly stimulatory effect, as well as a possible association with work if you're prone to checking emails while at home. Turning off digital devices and focusing on more passive and relaxing activities such as watching TV, reading or listening to music will help to calm the nervous system and help you to feel ready for bed.

Plenty of fresh air and exercise during the day can help to improve sleep, but avoid exercising too late in the evening as this can have a stimulatory effect which may increase your insomnia.

DID YOU KNOW?

Going to bed at the same time in the evening and getting up at the same time in the morning, even at weekends, can help to regulate your body clock so that your system becomes accustomed to the rhythm; this can make it easier to fall asleep and stay asleep.

3 Ways to Reduce Insomnia

1. Put all digital devices away at least an hour before bed and leave your phone outside the bedroom. Buy an alarm clock, if you usually use your phone to wake you up.
2. Avoid chocolate, crisps, biscuits and other sugary foods or alcohol in the evening as these will all disrupt blood sugar levels before bed.
3. Review your sleep environment so that you achieve the right temperature, level of darkness and quiet to suit you.

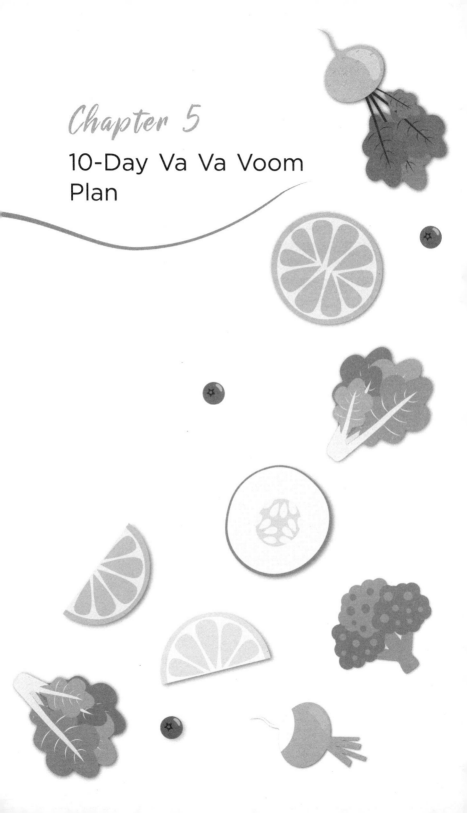

Chapter 5

10-Day Va Va Voom Plan

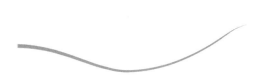

HOW THE PLAN WORKS

The Va Va Voom plan is modular so that you can choose the pace that suits you best by following either The Energiser Plan or The Super-Boost Plan.

WHICH PLAN IS RIGHT FOR ME?

The Energiser Plan takes a more gentle approach to help you adjust to the change of lifestyle by allowing a longer transition into and out of the plan and a shorter Cleansing phase. It's suitable for busy people who may find it difficult to implement some of the changes straight away or for people who feel that they may take some time to adjust to the new diet and lifestyle. The less intense pace would also be more appropriate if you're feeling extremely fatigued.

The Super-Boost Plan moves at a faster pace and allows less time to adjust to the change of lifestyle. The transition phases into and out of the programme are shorter and the Cleansing phase is extended. It's suitable for people who already follow a healthy diet and who feel they won't struggle with a sudden elimination of caffeine, sugar, wheat or alcohol.

The Energiser Plan Structure

Days 1, 2 and 3 are **Intro** Days – these are transition days to help ease you into the programme and wean you off energy-robbing anti-nutrients.

Days 4 and 5 are **Booster** Days – this is where the programme really starts to get going and the elimination will get a bit stricter.
Day 6 is a **Cleansing** Day – this is a fruit and vegetable day to cleanse the liver and ease any toxic burden on your body which might be compromising your energy levels. It's recommended to do this on a weekend day or another day when you're not working, so that you can take it easy.
Day 7 is another **Booster** Day – this should feel super-easy after the cleansing day.
Days 8, 9 and 10 are **Cruising** Days – you should be well into your stride by now, feeling far more energised. The Cruising Days ease off slightly from the Booster Days in preparation for the ongoing Maintenance Programme, which is the follow-up plan to encourage you to stick with your new healthy habits.

The Super-Boost Plan Structure

Day 1 is an **Intro** Day – this acts as a transition day to help ease you into the programme and wean you off anti-nutrients.
Days 2, 3 and 4 are **Booster** Days – this is where the programme really starts to get going and the elimination will get a bit stricter.
Days 5 and 6 are **Cleansing** Days – these are fruit and vege-table days to cleanse the liver and ease any toxic burden on your body. It's recommended to do this over a weekend or another two days when you're not working, so that you can take it easy. This phase could be extended to a third day if you're enjoying it and are feeling well. See FAQ number 8 (page 136).
Days 7 and 8 are **Booster** Days – these should feel super-easy after the cleansing days.
Days 9 and 10 are **Cruising** Days – you should be well into your stride by now, feeling far more energised. The Cruising Days ease off slightly from the Booster Days in preparation for the ongoing Maintenance Programme, which is the follow-up plan to encourage you to stick with your new healthy habits.

THE PRINCIPLES BEHIND THE 10-DAY VA VA VOOM PLAN

The Va Va Voom plan is based on 5 core principles:

1. Maintaining blood sugar balance

A blood sugar imbalance is one of the most common causes of low energy. Relying on sugar, refined carbohydrate or stimulants such as caffeine and alcohol for a quick burst of energy to keep you going can lead to a series of blood sugar highs and lows. Over the course of a day this can put a real strain on the body, and over time a blood sugar imbalance will not only lead to energy dips, but also insomnia at night and fatigue in the morning. If you tend to be pretty perky in the evening but are dragging yourself out of bed in the morning, the chances are that your blood sugar levels need some attention.

The biochemistry of blood sugar is explained in more detail on pages 78–9, but for the purpose of the plan, the key principles to remember are that you should eat protein and fibre with every meal and snack, eliminate sugary foods, refined carbohydrate, caffeine and alcohol and avoid long gaps between meals. The meals that feature in each stage of the plan are carefully designed examples of a blood sugar-balancing combination which you can follow or use as inspiration for planning your own meals.

Here are some examples of everyday foods that either help or hinder your blood sugar balance:

REFINED FOODS

- White bread
- White rice
- White pasta
- White noodles
- White couscous
- French fries
- Crisps
- Pizza
- Sugary breakfast cereal

HIGH-SUGAR FOODS

- Chocolate
- Biscuits
- Sweets
- Pastries and other baked goods
- Cakes
- Doughnuts
- Fizzy drinks
- Desserts
- Fruit juice
- Jams

COMMON SOURCES OF CAFFEINE

- Coffee
- Black tea; green tea; matcha tea; jasmine tea; white tea
- Cola
- Energy drinks and bars
- Chocolate
- Cold remedies and pain-killers

CAFFEINE-FREE OPTIONS

- Herbal infusions
- Water/sparkling water
- Rooibos/redbush tea
- Cordials and squash
- Decaffeinated coffee

GOOD SOURCES
OF PROTEIN

- Lean red meat
- White meat
- Fish
- Eggs
- Yoghurt
- Lentils
- Chickpeas/houmous
- Beans
- Nuts and seeds
- Quinoa

GOOD SOURCES
OF FIBRE

- Vegetables
- Fruit with edible skin
- Wholegrain bread
- Brown rice
- Oats
- Wholegrain pasta
- Pulses

2. Reducing inflammation

Chronic low-grade inflammation is increasingly recognised as one of the key underlying factors in a state of constant tiredness, which is why reducing inflammation is a key principle of the plan. Inflammation can manifest itself in lots of different ways, including joint or muscle pain; bloating and digestive discomfort; acne; eczema or dermatitis; headaches and sinusitis. It is also associated with a number of chronic health conditions. Inflammation is explained in more detail in Chapter 4.

Certain foods can activate inflammation in the body and others help to calm the inflammatory response, so the Va Va Voom plan aims to eliminate inflammatory foods and promote anti-inflammatory foods.

Here are some examples of everyday foods that are pro- or anti-inflammatory:

 PRO-INFLAMMATORY FOODS

- Wheat
- Refined carbohydrate
- Saturated fat
- Sugar
- Milk, cream and cheese
- Red meat
- Bacon, ham, salami
- Alcohol

ANTI-INFLAMMATORY FOODS

- Oily fish
- Vegetables
- Lentils, chickpeas, beans
- Fruit
- Nuts
- Seeds

Some grains are considered to be pro-inflammatory, but not every grain is eliminated in the Va Va Voom plan. Gluten is a protein which is found in wheat, rye and barley and which can cause inflammation in sensitive individuals. The Va Va Voom plan deliberately eliminates wheat rather than rye or barley because wheat features very strongly in many people's diet on a daily basis in the form of breakfast cereals, bread, pasta, noodles, baked goods and beer. Eliminating wheat for 10 days could provide a quick win in anti-inflammatory terms, helping to reduce the potential inflammatory load on the body, while still allowing for the flexibility of rye bread or rye crispbread to feature in the opening and closing stages of the programme.

COMMON FOODS THAT
CONTAIN WHEAT

- Most breads unless they're 100% rye or are made with gluten-free flour
- Pasta and noodles
- Couscous
- Biscuits
- Baked goods e.g. cakes, cookies, pastries
- Pie crusts, quiches, tarts
- Beer
- Soy sauce

WHEAT-FREE ALTERNATIVES

- Rye bread or crispbread
- Buckwheat breads, pancakes, pasta or noodles
- Millet breads or noodles
- Edamame, buckwheat or brown rice pasta
- Oats, rice or quinoa
- Tamari soy sauce

The Va Va Voom plan also applies a considered approach to dairy, which is another pro-inflammatory food group. Cow's milk and cheese tend to be the most inflammatory forms of dairy and these are eliminated throughout the 10 days. The opening and closing stages of the programme include natural yoghurt and cottage cheese; not only are these less inflammatory than standard milk or cheese, they also have other residual Va Va Voom-boosting benefits. Yoghurt contains beneficial bacteria which will support optimal gut function and promote nutrient absorption, and cottage cheese is a good source of protein, low in inflammatory saturated fat and contains some vitamin D.

COMMON FOODS THAT CONTAIN DAIRY

- Milk, butter, cheese, yoghurt, cream
- Batter and batter mixes
- Cakes, biscuits, pastries
- Most desserts

- Ice cream
- Chocolate
- White sauces

DAIRY-FREE ALTERNATIVES

- Almond milk
- Rice milk
- Soya milk, yoghurt or cheese
- Coconut milk, yoghurt or cheese
- Hazelnut milk

- Cashew milk or cheese
- Oat milk
- Olive, sunflower, avocado or coconut oil spreads
- Nut butters

3. Focusing on foods that contain Va Va Voom-boosting nutrients

The 10-day plan and the Maintenance Plan are specifically designed to feature a range of foods that will support your energy levels. The Va Va Voom quiz in Chapter 2 will have helped you to identify possible weak points in your energy production. You can use this information to personalise the plan so that you're focusing on the relevant Va Va Voom boosters for you. Take another look at Chapter 3 if you need a quick refresher.

By following the blood sugar-balancing advice above, you will naturally include sufficient Va Va Voom-boosting macronutrients. If you stick to the portion guidelines on page 131, you will ensure that you include enough vegetables, as these tend to be the best source of Va Va Voom micronutrients. Ensuring that at least 50% of your meal at lunch or dinner is made up of a variety of vegetables will also give your Va Va Voom a huge boost.

4. Eliminating Va Va Voom-robbing food and drink from your diet

Most of the Va Va Voom-robbing food and drink will probably come as no surprise, as the list includes refined sugar, alcohol, caffeine, wheat and processed food. All of these will disrupt the energy-production process in the body either directly or indirectly which is why they've been removed from the 10-day plan. The information in Chapter 4 includes some background explanation and justification that may help you to keep up your motivation as you work through the 10-day plan.

5. Va Va Voom-boosting wellbeing activities

It's important to factor in time for wellbeing activities which will support your quest for Va Va Voom. Research has shown that exercise, mindfulness, relaxation activities and improved quality of sleep all have a very positive effect on energy levels. The Wellbeing Wheel has been designed to make sure that you don't neglect this really important element of the plan. Committing to 2 actions from each section of the wheel during the programme will make a big difference to the way you feel at the end of the 10 days.

HOW TO PREPARE FOR YOUR 10-DAY VA VA VOOM PLAN

Get Yourself in Training

It's always wise to ease yourself gently into a change of diet and lifestyle so that it's not too much of a shock to the system. If caffeine, alcohol, sugar or processed foods feature regularly in your diet, it would be a very smart move to gradually reduce them during the week before you start the Va Va Voom plan. The addictive nature of this type of food and drink can mean some unpleasant withdrawal symptoms, such as headaches, tiredness or aching joints. You'll gain a lot more benefit from the plan and find it much easier if you've had a bit of a clean-up before you get started.

The plan is designed to start on a Monday, so that the Cleansing Days fall at the weekend. As these days can be a little challenging, it's best if you're able to be at home and take things slowly, so that it doesn't feel too overwhelming. Of course, you can start the programme whenever it suits you if your working week follows a different pattern or if you want to manage things differently.

Give Your Kitchen Cupboard a Makeover

Give yourself the best possible chance of avoiding the temptation that often lurks in your kitchen cupboard by having a good clear-out. Get rid of any biscuits, cake, chocolate, sweets, crisps or sugary cereals and make sure there isn't a stray can of beer or bottle of wine lying around as this may only make it harder for you to stick to your new regime.

If this is likely to cause uproar amongst the rest of the household and you're the person in charge of the shopping, then stock the house with brands or products that you actively dislike. It'll make it a lot easier to walk away!

Go Shopping

Here are some staple foods that you might find useful to stock up on as you're likely to be using them regularly throughout the plan. Where possible, according to availability and your budget, opt for organic products – the use of pesticides, fungicides, hormones and antibiotics is closely regulated, which will reduce the potential toxic load of the foods.

Store cupboard

Quinoa
Brown rice
Oats
Rough oatcakes or brown rice cakes
Wheat-free pasta or noodles
Chickpeas
Low-sugar baked beans
Red lentils
Puy lentils
Olive oil

Rapeseed oil
Red wine vinegar
Apple cider vinegar
Balsamic vinegar
Maple syrup
Tuna in spring water
Arrabbiata or puttanesca pasta sauce
Vegetable stock
Tamari wheat-free soy sauce
An additive-free protein powder e.g. pea, rice or soy
Pumpkin seeds
Sunflower seeds
Mixed nuts (walnuts, almonds, hazelnuts)
Tinned tomatoes
Herbal teas
Cordials

Dairy free

Unsweetened almond, soya, oat, rice, hazelnut, cashew or
   coconut milk
Sunflower, olive or avocado oil dairy-free spread
Unsweetened peanut, almond, cashew or pumpkin seed butter
Coconut or soya milk yoghurts
Cashew or soya cheese

Fresh

Houmous (full-fat)
Cottage cheese (full-fat)
Natural yoghurt (full-fat)
Eggs
100% rye bread (check the label for added wheat flour because
   some manufacturers use a wheat/rye blend)
Parsley
Basil
Coriander
Thyme
Rosemary

Frozen

> Frozen blueberries or raspberries (a cost-effective and healthy
>   option and very handy for making smoothies)
> Spinach
> Peas

If you can't find what you're looking for in a local supermarket or
health food store, here are some useful online suppliers that are a
one-stop shop for healthy foods and that stock a range of brands.

www.goodnessdirect.co.uk
www.healthysupplies.co.uk
www.buywholefoodsonline.co.uk

HOW TO MANAGE YOUR 10-DAY VA VA VOOM PLAN

Structure Your Day Carefully

Make sure that you have a meal or small snack roughly every 3–4
hours. Your day might look like this:

7am	10am	1pm	4pm	7pm
Breakfast	Snack	Lunch	Snack	Dinner

Or like this if you have a late breakfast or tend to stay late at work:

9am	12pm	3pm	6pm	9pm
Breakfast	Lunch	Snack	Snack	Dinner

Avoid long gaps between meals as this can lead to a drop in blood
sugar, making you feel tired and irritable. You don't have to eat a
snack if you don't feel hungry, but it's important to make sure that
you don't allow your blood sugar to drop dramatically between
meals. If your energy levels drop, you'll crave sugary foods and

refined carbohydrate, which might provide a quick fix but will lead to an energy crash later in the day.

Manage Your Portions Correctly

For breakfast, please follow the guidelines set out in the meal planner. For lunch and dinner, protein and starch should each represent 25% of the overall meal, (aim for a portion about the size of your fist for each) and vegetables should make up 50% of the meal. If you're not eating starch at a meal, increase the vegetable portion to 75% of the overall meal. Following these proportions will support your blood sugar and ensure optimum levels of Va Va Voom-boosting foods.

The Va Va Voom Plate

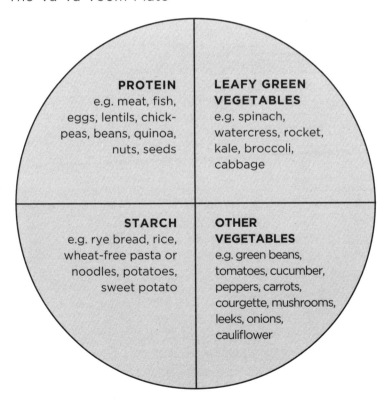

NB: it's **very important** *not to stint on the vegetable portion, as they are such an important part of the energy equation.*

THE 10-DAY VA VA VOOM PLAN FAQS

1. What can I eat on the different days?

	PROTEIN	STARCH
Intro Days	Meat, fish, eggs, natural yoghurt, dairy-free milk, cottage cheese, quinoa, lentils, chickpeas, houmous, falafel, beans, nuts, seeds	Brown rice, brown rice cakes, oats, rough oatcakes, 100% rye bread, rye crispbread, wheat-free pasta, new potatoes, sweet potato, quinoa, pulses
Booster Days	Meat, fish, eggs, quinoa, lentils, chickpeas, houmous, falafel, beans, nuts, seeds, dairy-free milk	Brown rice, quinoa, oats, pulses
Cleansing Days	Nuts, seeds	N/A
Cruising Days	Meat, fish, eggs, natural yoghurt, dairy-free milk, cottage cheese, quinoa, lentils, chickpeas, houmous, falafel, beans, nuts, seeds	Brown rice, brown rice cakes, oats, rough oatcakes, 100% rye bread, rye crispbread, new potatoes, sweet potato, quinoa, pulses

VEGETABLES	FRUIT	DRINKS
All	All	Water, herbal tea, freshly squeezed fruit or veg juice (no carton products), recommended smoothies (see recipes), caffeine-free tea or coffee
All except potatoes and sweet potato	All	Water, herbal tea, freshly squeezed fruit or veg juice (no carton products), recommended smoothies (see recipes)
All except potatoes and sweet potato	All	Water, herbal tea, freshly squeezed fruit or veg juice (no carton products), recommended smoothies (see recipes)
All	All	Water, herbal tea, freshly squeezed fruit or veg juice (no carton products), recommended smoothies (see recipes)

2. Should I only eat the recommended meals?

The meal planners are there to provide guidance and inspiration. There are plenty of different options to allow for variety throughout the 10 days, but you're completely free to use some of your own favourite recipes if you'd prefer to do that. All you need to do is to make sure that the different ingredients you use fall within the guidelines for whichever part of the plan you're following and that you stick to the basic principle of combining protein- and fibre-rich foods.

3. Can I have dessert?

Most desserts are pretty sugary and therefore likely to disrupt all the careful choices you've made with your main meals so they're best avoided for the next 10 days. A small piece of fresh fruit could be an option, but if you have sluggish digestion or struggle with symptoms of bloating and wind, it's best to eat fruit at least 2 hours away from a meal as this can make things worse. Fruit breaks down very quickly in the body and may start to ferment as it waits for the rest of the meal to digest, which can lead to digestive discomfort. One or two squares of very dark chocolate (80%+) is a great low-sugar option or you could consider a sweet herbal tea, such as liquorice, vanilla or mixed fruit, as this can help to take the edge off cravings for sweet things.

4. Why do you recommend full-fat products?

It's important to avoid the low-fat trap. A common misconception is that foods containing fat are bad for you, which is far from the case. Dietary fat is a crucial part of our diet – mono-unsaturated and polyunsaturated fats are essential for heart, brain and hormone health, while saturated fat helps to make sex hormones and stores essential energy-boosting nutrients such as vitamin D. Fat is also a rich source of energy for the body. Low-fat products usually contain higher levels of sugar or salt to make up for the loss of flavour that comes from stripping out the fat.

5. Should I limit the amount of eggs I eat?

Eggs are practically a superfood! They're packed with protein and the yolk is full of energy-boosting vitamins and minerals. The yolk also contains cholesterol which is why eggs have had a bad press in the past. However, repeated studies have demonstrated that dietary cholesterol does not impact levels of cholesterol in our blood. Eggs are highly nutritious and there is no recommended limit on how many we should eat. However, a balanced and healthy diet is all about variety, so it would be sensible to avoid eating eggs at every meal, to make sure that you're having a range of different sources of nutrients across the day.

6. Does it matter if I skip the Intro Days?

It's always wise to introduce big changes to your diet in a gradual way. This allows your body to make the transition more easily and can help to avoid any unpleasant withdrawal symptoms that may occur when you eliminate addictive elements such as caffeine or sugar. Rushing into dietary changes or applying an overly strict regime can often make it more difficult to stick to a diet plan after about 3 days. The Va Va Voom plans are carefully designed to be achievable and sustainable, so it's best to follow the structure that is laid out, whichever plan you chose.

7. How much water should I drink?

Hydration is highly individual and will depend on your height, weight, level of physical activity and whether you live or work in a hot environment. As we've seen in Chapter 4, even mild dehydration can significantly affect energy, productivity and performance. Aim for 6–8 glasses per day if you have a moderately active lifestyle and increase it according to the factors listed above if you display any of the signs of dehydration listed in Chapter 4. This can include cordials and squash, sparkling water, herbal teas and vegetable juices as well as plain water.

8. Can I do more of the Cleansing Days if I want to?

If you've chosen to do The Energiser Plan, you should stick with the recommended 1 Cleansing Day, as the plan is carefully structured to support people with a hectic lifestyle or who want to take things gently. You can always try The Super-Boost Plan at a later date if you want to extend the Cleansing Days.

If you've chosen to do The Super-Boost Plan, you could do 3 Cleansing Days instead of 2, if you're enjoying it, feeling good and know that it won't put too much pressure on you. You can follow this with 2 Booster Days and 1 Cruising Day to help your body adjust before you move on to the Maintenance Plan. It's important not to do any more than 3 Cleansing Days on this programme and make sure you're not adding in the extra day out of a misplaced sense of competitiveness. Two days will be more than enough for you to achieve your Va Va Voom goals.

9. Will I lose weight on the plan?

The Va Va Voom plan is not designed to be a weight-loss diet, but you may well find that you lose a few pounds along the way. Many of the Va Va Voom robbers that are eliminated from your diet during the 10 days are typically foods that encourage weight gain, so some weight loss may be an additional benefit if your diet normally contains a lot of sugar, bread or alcohol, for example. The increased level of activity promoted by the Wellbeing Wheel could also kick-start weight loss if you have a sedentary lifestyle. As the programme progresses you're likely to feel more energised and motivated to exercise, which may also improve body tone.

10. Can I repeat the plan when I've finished it?

The 10-day plan isn't designed to be followed consistently. When you finish, it's best to move on to the Maintenance Plan. This plan takes a more sustainable approach and you can adapt it to include your learnings from the 10-day plan, to help you build a personalised Va Va Voom diet and lifestyle. If you'd like a Va Va Voom boost from time to time, schedule in a 10-day plan once a quarter to help you keep on track.

11. Should I check with my doctor before starting the plan?

If you have any medical conditions or are taking any medication, you should always check in with your doctor before making any drastic changes to your diet and lifestyle.

THE 10-DAY VA VA VOOM PLAN

The Energiser Plan	The Super-Boost Plan
Days 1–3 – Intro Days	**Day 1 – Intro Day**

Welcome to the Intro Days. These days are carefully designed to help you get into the Va Va Voom zone by providing a gentle transition from your everyday diet. You'll start to eliminate some key elements of your diet that could be sapping your energy. The Intro Days are free from wheat, caffeine, alcohol, refined sugar and processed foods. They're also mostly dairy free. Read the guideline section below for the full details.

INTRO DAY GUIDELINES

- Eat a combination of protein and fibre with every meal and snack
- Enjoy rye bread maximum once a day
- Enjoy either new potatoes or sweet potato maximum once a day
- Eat at least 2 handfuls of raw or cooked leafy greens such as spinach, watercress, cabbage, broccoli and kale per day
- It's time to eliminate alcohol, caffeine, refined sugar, processed foods and wheat from your diet, but there are still plenty of great-tasting options left!
- Eliminate cow's milk and cheese; enjoy goat's or sheep's cheese maximum once a day; enjoy cottage cheese
- Limit your intake of red meat to twice a week
- Drink plenty of water or herbal teas

WHAT CAN I EAT ON AN INTRO DAY?

ENJOY (eat throughout the day)	LIMIT (follow the restrictions in the guidelines)	ELIMINATE
Beans Brown rice or brown rice crackers Chickpeas Cottage cheese Dairy-free milks Eggs Fruit Houmous Lentils Natural yoghurt Nuts Oats or oatcakes Oily fish, white fish Quinoa Rye crispbread Seeds Vegetables White meat	Goat's and sheep's cheese Lean red meat New potatoes and sweet potato 100% rye bread (check label for any wheat flour) Wheat-free pasta	Alcohol Baked goods e.g. cakes, cookies, pastries, muffins, pies, tarts Caffeine Chocolate, confectionery and crisps Cow's milk and cheese (except for cottage cheese) Dried fruit Ice cream Potatoes (except new potatoes and sweet potato) Processed meat e.g. all ham, salami, bacon Sugar and sugary foods Wheat e.g. pasta, noodles, couscous, bread, some breakfast cereals

MEAL PLANNER FOR INTRO DAYS

The meal planner is designed to provide some helpful guidance and inspiration as you work through each phase. Anything that is flagged with the letter R will feature in the recipes in Chapter 7.

BREAKFAST	Eggs
A combination of protein- and fibre-rich foods is the best way to ensure sustained energy throughout the morning and to avoid cravings for energy-robbing foods. Choose one of these options or create your own breakfast, following the Va Va Voom protein–fibre principle explained on page 81.	• 1–2 poached, scrambled or boiled eggs with 1–2 slices of rye toast and dairy-free spread (use olive oil to scramble the eggs) • 1–2 poached or scrambled eggs with wilted spinach and fried mushrooms • Vegetable omelette (R) • 1–2 poached eggs with ½ an avocado or smoked salmon with 1–2 slices of rye toast and dairy-free spread
LUNCH	Soup
Avoiding large portions of starchy carbohydrate at lunchtime will help to prevent the dreaded mid-afternoon slump. Baguette sandwiches, jacket potatoes or large portions of rice and pasta are likely to have you nodding off by 3pm! Remember to include plenty of protein with your lunch, as this will keep you going for longer.	• Lentil & tomato soup (R) with (optional) 1 slice of rye bread • Herby bean soup (R) with (optional) 1 slice of rye bread • Lemony chicken & vegetable soup (R) with (optional) 1 slice of rye bread

Grains	Fruit & Veg	Quick & Easy
• Overnight oats with dairy-free milk, fresh fruit and mixed seeds (R) • 40–50g of homemade granola (R) with natural yoghurt and blueberries • Classic porridge with dairy-free milk, berries and chopped walnuts (R) • Quinoa porridge with dairy-free milk and raspberries (R)	• Vitality smoothie (R) • Gorgeous green smoothie (R) • Breakfast smoothie (R) • Fresh fruit salad with nuts, seeds and natural yoghurt (R)	• Unsweetened peanut, cashew or almond butter with 1–2 slices of rye toast (if you don't eat nuts, try a protein-rich seed butter such as pumpkin seed butter)
Salad	**Hot Meal**	**Quick & Easy**
Use the Va Va Voom Salad Bar on page 220 to help you construct your own salad e.g. • Quinoa & avocado salad (R) • Butternut squash & feta salad (R) • Smoked mackerel & beetroot salad (R)	• Jacket sweet potato with cottage cheese and spinach salad • Vegetable omelette (R) • Courgette & pea frittata (R) with tomato & rocket salad • Chicken with brown rice and stir-fried vegetables (R)	• Rye bread sandwich with tuna mayo, cucumber & tomato • Rye bread sandwich with egg & cress • Rye bread sandwich with houmous, spinach & tomato

DINNER	Meat
A careful combination of protein- and fibre-rich food will help to ensure blood sugar balance before bedtime, setting you up for a good night's sleep. Remember to follow the Va Va Voom Plate diagram to get the portions right.	• Steak with sweet potato fries (R), peas and roasted cherry tomatoes • Grilled chicken with mixed salad (R) • Shepherd's pie with crushed new potato topping (R)
SNACKS	Fruit & Nuts/Seeds
If you tend to leave very long gaps between meals, a small snack will help to maintain energy levels and ensure that you arrive at the next meal hungry, rather than desperate. This will ensure you choose long-term energy-boosting foods rather than grabbing a carby quick fix. Make sure every snack includes some form of protein!	• 1 apple, clementine, plum or other fruit with an edible skin PLUS 7–8 raw, unsalted almonds, walnuts or hazelnuts • 7–8 rosemary-roasted almonds (R) NB: if nuts don't work for you, try munching on a tablespoon of pumpkin or sunflower seeds instead
DRINKS	Juice
Remember that just 2% dehydration can affect energy levels by up to 15%. Keeping yourself nicely topped up with fluid throughout the day in whichever form suits you best will definitely increase your Va Va Voom.	• Avoid pure fruit juices, especially anything in a carton as these will send your blood sugar soaring. • Opt for freshly squeezed vegetable juices with just a small amount of fruit to sweeten it.

Fish	Vegetarian	Quick & Easy
• Salmon with lentils and garlic-roasted vegetables (R) • Prawn & pak choi stir fry (R) • Roasted haddock with citrus rice (R)	• Quinoa with garlic-roasted vegetables (R) • Vegetable & bean chilli with brown rice (R) • Lentil & vegetable casserole (R)	• Wheat-free pasta with a small can of tuna or 120g of cooked prawns with ½ 350g jar of puttanesca or arrabbiata tomato sauce • 200g of low-sugar baked beans on rye toast with dairy-free spread

Oat or Rice Cakes	Vegetables	Cereal Bar or Ball
• 1–2 rough oatcakes or brown rice cakes with 50g houmous, unsweetened nut butter or cottage cheese	• A handful of carrot, celery, pepper or cucumber sticks with 50g of houmous, cottage cheese or guacamole • Pea power smoothie (R) • 15g of spicy roasted chickpeas (R)	Opt for something that contains plenty of nuts and seeds for a protein boost. Beware of sugary cereal bars, especially anything with large amounts of dried fruit (dates are commonly used to sweeten health bars and are very high in sugar).

Hot drinks	Water	Squash or cordial
• Herbal infusions such as peppermint, camomile, fennel or liquorice tea • Fruit teas • Rooibos/redbush tea (caffeine free) • Decaffeinated coffee	• Still and sparkling water • Coconut water (don't have more than 330ml per day because it can contain a lot of fruit sugar)	Where possible opt for low-sugar options. Try out interesting new flavours such as elderflower, ginger or raspberry. Added to sparkling water they make a lovely drink with a celebratory feel.

The Energiser Plan   The Super-Boost Plan

Days 4-5 - Booster Days   Days 2-4 - Booster Days

Congratulations on completing the Intro phase of the plan. You're now ready to move to the Booster Days. This is where you'll build on the progress you made in the first few days and start to eliminate some of the other potential energy robbers in your diet so that you're all set to start your cleanse in a few days' time. The Booster Days exclude wheat, dairy, alcohol, caffeine and refined sugar. Pay careful attention to the guidelines below to make sure that you're keeping on track, especially with the foods in the Limit column.

BOOSTER DAY GUIDELINES

- Eat a combination of protein and fibre with every meal and snack
- Eat at least 2 handfuls of raw or cooked leafy greens like spinach, watercress, rocket, cabbage and kale per day
- It's time to eliminate all dairy, including natural yoghurt, cottage cheese, goat's and sheep's milk and cheese
- Eliminate all bread and pasta, including rye bread and rye crispbread and wheat-free pasta
- Continue to eliminate alcohol, caffeine, refined sugar, wheat and processed foods
- Limit your intake of red meat to twice a week
- Eat rice, rice cakes or oatcakes maximum once a day
- Enjoy all vegetables except potatoes and sweet potato and make sure you hit your vegetable-portion target at lunch and dinner
- Focus on fruits with an edible skin as they are higher in fibre and lower in sugar – limit sweet fleshy fruit such as mango, pineapple, banana and grapes to maximum once a day
- Vary your fruit throughout the day so that you only have one portion of each type of fruit e.g. 1 apple, 1 satsuma, 1 portion of blueberries etc

WHAT CAN I EAT ON A BOOSTER DAY?

ENJOY (eat throughout the day)	LIMIT (follow the restrictions in the guidelines)	ELIMINATE
Beans Chickpeas Dairy-free milk or yoghurt Eggs Falafel Fruit with edible skin Houmous Lentils Nuts and nut butters Oily fish, white fish Quinoa Seeds and seed butters Vegetables White meat	Brown rice, brown rice cakes Sweet fleshy fruit e.g. mango, pineapple, banana, grapes Oats, rough oatcakes Lean red meat	Alcohol Baked goods e.g. cakes, cookies, pastries, muffins, pies, tarts All bread, rye crispbread, pasta, noodles, couscous Caffeine Chocolate and confectionery All cow's, goat's and sheep's milk, yoghurt and cheese, including cottage cheese Dried fruit Ice cream Potatoes, sweet potato Processed meat e.g. ham, salami, bacon Sugar and sugary foods

MEAL PLANNER FOR BOOSTER DAYS

BREAKFAST	Eggs
A combination of protein- and fibre-rich food is the best way to ensure sustained energy throughout the morning and to avoid cravings for energy-robbing foods. Choose one of these options or create your own breakfast, following the Va Va Voom protein–fibre principle explained on page 81.	• 1–2 scrambled or poached eggs with wilted spinach and fried mushrooms (use olive oil to scramble the eggs) • Vegetable omelette (R) • 1–2 poached eggs with sliced avocado
LUNCH	Soup
Avoiding large portions of starchy carbohydrate at lunchtime will help to prevent the dreaded mid-afternoon slump. Baguette sandwiches, jacket potatoes or large portions of rice and pasta are likely to have you nodding off by 3pm! Remember to include plenty of protein with your lunch, as this will keep you going for longer.	• Lentil & tomato soup (R) with (optional) 2 rough oatcakes or brown rice cakes • Herby bean soup (R) with (optional) 2 rough oatcakes or brown rice cakes • Lemony chicken & vegetable soup (R) with (optional) 2 rough oatcakes or brown rice cakes

Grains	Fruit & Veg	Quick & Easy
• Overnight oats with dairy-free milk, fresh fruit and mixed seeds (R) • 40–50g of homemade granola (R) with natural yoghurt and blueberries • Classic porridge with dairy-free milk, berries and chopped walnuts (R) • Quinoa porridge with dairy-free milk and raspberries (R)	• Overnight oats smoothie (R) • Pea power smoothie (R) • Booster juice (R) with 1 tablespoon of pea, rice or soy protein powder (no additives or sugar) • Fresh fruit salad with nuts & seeds (R) and soya or coconut milk yoghurt	• 1 apple with 50g of unsweetened peanut, cashew or almond butter

Salad	Hot Meal	Quick & Easy
Use the Va Va Voom Salad Bar on page 220 to help you construct your own salad e.g. • Quinoa & avocado salad (R) • Prawn salad with brown rice and Asian dressing (R) • Smoked mackerel & beetroot salad	• Vegetable omelette (R) • Courgette & pea frittata (R) with tomato & rocket salad • Chicken with brown rice and stir-fried vegetables (R)	• Pre-cooked chicken breast or pre-poached salmon with ½ a bag of salad leaves, tomato and cucumber • 4 rough oatcakes or brown rice cakes with 50g houmous, chopped carrot sticks and an apple

DINNER	Meat
A careful combination of protein- and fibre-rich food will help to ensure blood sugar balance before bedtime, setting you up for a good night's sleep. Remember to follow the Va Va Voom Plate diagram on page 131 to get the portions right.	• Grilled steak with citrus rice (R), broccoli and roasted tomatoes • Grilled chicken with cauliflower rice, spinach and roasted red vegetables (R) • Oven-baked venison sausages (R) with garlic-roasted vegetables (R)

SNACKS	Fruit & Nuts/Seeds
If you tend to leave long gaps between meals, a small snack will help to maintain your energy levels and ensure that you arrive at the next meal hungry, rather than desperate. This will ensure you choose sustaining energy-boosting foods rather than grabbing a carby quick fix. Make sure every snack includes some form of protein!	• 1 apple, clementine, plum or other fruit with an edible skin PLUS 7–8 raw unsalted almonds, walnuts or hazelnuts, or 1 tablespoon of pumpkin or sunflower seeds • 7–8 rosemary-roasted almonds (R) with an apple • A small pot of plain coconut or soya yoghurt with a tablespoon of fresh blueberries

DRINKS	Juice
Remember that just 2% dehydration can affect energy levels by up to 15%. Keeping yourself nicely topped up with fluid throughout the day in whichever form suits you best will definitely increase your Va Va Voom.	• Avoid pure fruit juices, especially anything in a carton, as these will send your blood sugar soaring. • Opt for freshly squeezed vegetable juices with just a small amount of fruit to sweeten it.

Fish	Vegetarian	Quick & Easy
• Salmon with lentils and garlic-roasted vegetables (R) • Prawn & pak choi stir fry (R) • Roasted haddock with citrus rice (R)	• Quinoa with garlic-roasted vegetables (R) • Vegetable & bean chilli with brown rice (R) • Lentil & vegetable casserole (R)	• 200g of low-sugar baked beans with grilled venison sausages

Oat or Rice Cakes	Vegetables	Cereal Bar or Ball
• 1-2 rough oatcakes or brown rice cakes with houmous, unsweetened nut butter or guacamole	• A handful of carrot, celery, pepper or cucumber sticks with 50g of houmous, or guacamole • Summer cup juice (R) • 15g of spicy roasted chickpeas (R)	Opt for something that contains plenty of nuts or seeds for a protein boost. Beware of sugary cereal bars, especially anything with large amounts of dried fruit (dates, are commonly used to sweeten health bars and are very high in sugar).

Hot drinks	Water	Squash or cordial
• Herbal infusions such as peppermint, camomile, fennel or liquorice tea • Fruit teas • Rooibos/redbush tea (caffeine free) • Decaffeinated coffee	• Still and sparkling water • Coconut water (don't have more than 330ml per day because it can contain a lot of fruit sugar)	Where possible opt for low-sugar options. Try out interesting new flavours such as elderflower, ginger or raspberry. Added to sparkling water they make a lovely drink with a celebratory feel.

The Energiser Plan   The Super-Boost Plan

Day 6 – Cleansing Day   Days 5-6 – Cleansing Days

It's time to get serious! Over the past few days you've removed a lot of potential energy robbers from your diet, which should make it much easier to carry out the Cleansing Day. Remember to take it easy – you need to be kind to yourself on a Cleansing Day. It's a perfect opportunity for a massage or other relaxing activity. This is a fruit-and-vegetable day with the option of a few nuts and seeds to support protein levels.

CLEANSING DAY GUIDELINES

- Eat fresh fruit, vegetables, herbs and spices only; eliminate all other foods except for a small amount of raw nuts, seeds and avocado (see below)
- At least 50% of the fruit and vegetables should be raw
- Aim to have no more than 4 portions of fruit across the day and make sure they're varied
- If you feel you need a quick protein boost eat 25g of nuts and seeds maximum per day
- Eat a maximum of one avocado per day
- Drink plenty of water throughout the day – at least 6–8 glasses
- A maximum of 2 tablespoons of oil (olive or rapeseed) per day are allowed to liven up your salads or for cooking vegetables

---

WHAT CAN I EAT ON A CLEANSING DAY?

ENJOY (eat throughout the day)	LIMIT (follow the restrictions in the guidelines)	ELIMINATE
Vegetables Fruit Herbs Spices Water Herbal tea	Raw nuts and seeds (25g maximum per day) Avocado Olive or rapeseed oil (2 tablespoons maximum per day)	Alcohol Baked goods e.g. cakes, cookies, pastries, muffins, pies, tarts All bread, rye crispbread, pasta, noodles, couscous Caffeine Chocolate and confectionery All cow's, goat's and sheep's milk, yoghurt and cheese Dried fruit Grains e.g. wheat, rice, oats, quinoa Ice cream Meat, fish, eggs, lentils, chickpeas, beans Potatoes, sweet potato, butternut squash Processed meat e.g. ham, salami, bacon Sugar and sugary foods

HOW TO SURVIVE THE CLEANSING DAY

- Try to schedule it over a weekend, preferably choosing a quiet time when you're mostly at home, not distracted by work and can take it relatively easy. Even though it is only a 1- or 2-day cleanse, it may seem very challenging, so ensure you choose a time when you're not pushing yourself too hard.
- Plan your shopping in advance to ensure you have all the appropriate ingredients to hand. If you have to shop in the middle of the cleanse, it's very tempting to pick up foods that you're trying to eliminate.
- Remove anything from the house that may be a temptation.
- Make sure you have a properly balanced meal the night before, so that you don't go into the cleanse feeling starving!
- Blood sugar management is important during the cleanse, as you'll be eating limited protein on this day. Eat more vegetables than fruit, as this will support fibre levels, and focus on eating whole raw fruit rather than fruit juices. Pure fruit juices will be very quickly absorbed by the body, giving a sugar boost, which could lead to blood sugar swings.
- Eat your fruit and vegetables slowly and mindfully. This will help you really make the most of what you're eating. The chewing process helps to activate our satiety response which tells us when we're full.
- Try to eat little and often to avoid getting too hungry, as it will be harder to commit to the cleanse if you leave long gaps between eating.
- Treat yourself throughout the day with relaxing activities you enjoy: a luxurious bath, a walk in the park or a massage. Keep yourself occupied with non-strenuous activities, so that you won't be tempted to break the cleanse.

MEAL PLANNER FOR CLEANSING DAYS

The timings below aren't fixed but are simply designed to give you an idea of how you can graze throughout the day to keep yourself going. You don't have to eat if you're not feeling hungry, but it's important not to leave long gaps between eating as this will make the day much harder for you.

8am	• Pea power smoothie (R) or • Fruit & veg platter with 15g of sunflower or pumpkin seeds or raw nuts (R)
10am	• Carrot, celery or cucumber sticks or • Tomato and carrot juice (R)
11.30am	• 10g of pumpkin seeds and 1 satsuma or • Booster juice (R)
1pm	• Spicy green & red salad with tomato salsa (R) or • Garlic-roasted vegetables (R) or • Tomato & basil soup (R)
3pm	• Vitality smoothie (R) or • 1 apple and 10g of raw almonds or walnuts
5pm	• 15g of spicy roasted chickpeas (R) or • 1 satsuma
Dinner	• Mixed vegetable salad with spicy salsa (R) or • Broccoli & sage soup (R)
Drinks	Drinking plenty of water, cordials, juice or herbal teas throughout the day is especially important on the Cleansing Days. As well as supporting the elimination of toxins, drinking plenty of fluid will help you feel energised during this more challenging phase of the programme.

The Energiser Plan   The Super-Boost Plan

Day 7 – Booster Day   Days 7–8 – Booster Days

Congratulations! Having completed your cleanse you should be feeling clear-headed and energised. Returning to another Booster Day is going to feel like a walk in the park in comparison! It's time to enjoy all the different available food choices. Remember that the Booster Days are still free from wheat, dairy, alcohol, caffeine, processed foods and refined sugar. Pay careful attention to the guidelines below to make sure that you're keeping on track, especially with the foods in the Limit column.

BOOSTER DAY GUIDELINES

- You can now reintroduce meat, fish, eggs, pulses and quinoa, which will help you stick to a combination of protein and fibre with meals and snacks
- Eat brown rice, brown rice cakes or oatcakes maximum once a day
- Eat at least 2 handfuls of raw or cooked leafy greens like spinach, watercress, rocket, cabbage and kale per day
- Continue to eliminate alcohol, caffeine, refined sugar, wheat and processed foods
- Continue to eliminate dairy, including natural yoghurt, cottage cheese, goat's and sheep's milk and cheese
- Continue to eliminate bread and pasta, including rye bread, rye crispbread and wheat-free pasta
- Limit red meat to a maximum of twice a week
- Enjoy all vegetables except potatoes, sweet potato and butternut squash and make sure you hit your vegetable-portion target at lunch and dinner
- Focus on fruits with an edible skin as they are higher in fibre and lower in sugar – limit sweet fleshy fruit such as mango, pineapple, banana and grapes to maximum once a day
- Vary your fruit throughout the day so that you only have one portion of each type e.g. 1 apple, 1 satsuma, 1 portion of blueberries etc.

WHAT CAN I EAT ON A BOOSTER DAY?

ENJOY (eat throughout the day)	LIMIT (follow the restrictions in the guidelines)	ELIMINATE
Beans Chickpeas Dairy-free milk or yoghurt Eggs Falafel Fruit with edible skin Houmous Lentils Nuts and nut butters Oily fish, white fish Quinoa Seeds and seed butters Vegetables White meat	Brown rice, brown rice cakes Sweet fleshy fruit e.g. mango, pineapple, banana, grapes Oats, rough oatcakes Lean red meat	Alcohol Baked goods e.g. cakes, cookies, pastries, muffins, pies, tarts All bread, rye crispbread, pasta, noodles, couscous Caffeine Chocolate and confectionery All cow's, goat's and sheep's milk, yoghurt and cheese, including cottage cheese Dried fruit Ice cream Potatoes, sweet potato Processed meat e.g. ham, salami, bacon Sugar and sugary foods

MEAL PLANNER FOR BOOSTER DAYS

BREAKFAST	Eggs
A combination of protein- and fibre-rich food is the best way to ensure sustained energy throughout the morning and to avoid cravings for energy-robbing foods. Choose one of these options or create your own breakfast, following the Va Va Voom protein–fibre principle explained on page 81.	• 1–2 scrambled or poached eggs with wilted spinach and fried mushrooms (use olive oil to scramble the eggs) • Vegetable omelette (R) • 1–2 poached eggs with sliced avocado
LUNCH	**Soup**
Avoiding large portions of starchy carbohydrate at lunchtime will help to prevent the dreaded mid-afternoon slump. Baguette sandwiches, jacket potatoes or large portions of rice and pasta are likely to have you nodding off by 3pm! Remember to include plenty of protein with your lunch, as this will keep you going for longer.	• Lentil & tomato soup (R) with (optional) 2 rough oatcakes or brown rice cakes • Herby bean soup (R) with (optional) 2 rough oatcakes or brown rice cakes • Lemony chicken & vegetable soup (R) with (optional) 2 rough oatcakes or brown rice cakes

Grains	Fruit & Veg	Quick & Easy
• Overnight oats with dairy-free milk, fresh fruit and mixed seeds (R) • 40–50g of homemade granola (R) with natural yoghurt and blueberries • Classic porridge with dairy-free milk, berries and chopped walnuts (R) • Quinoa porridge with dairy-free milk and raspberries (R)	• Overnight oats smoothie (R) • Pea power smoothie (R) • Booster juice (R) with 1 tablespoon of pea, rice or soy protein powder (no additives or sugar) • Fresh fruit salad with nuts & seeds (R) and soya or coconut milk yoghurt	• 1 apple with 50g of unsweetened peanut, cashew or almond butter
Salad	**Hot Meal**	**Quick & Easy**
Use the Va Va Voom Salad Bar on page 220 to help you construct your own salad e.g. • Quinoa & avocado salad (R) • Prawn salad with brown rice and Asian dressing (R) • Smoked mackerel & beetroot salad (R)	• Vegetable omelette (R) • Courgette & pea frittata (R) with tomato & rocket salad • Chicken with brown rice and stir-fried vegetables (R)	• Pre-cooked chicken breast or pre-poached salmon with ½ a bag of salad leaves, tomato and cucumber • 4 rough oatcakes or brown rice cakes with 50g houmous, chopped carrot sticks and an apple

DINNER	Meat
A careful combination of protein- and fibre-rich food will help to ensure blood sugar balance before bedtime, setting you up for a good night's sleep. Remember to follow the Va Va Voom Plate diagram on page 131 to get the portions right.	• Grilled steak with citrus rice (R), broccoli and roasted tomatoes • Grilled chicken with cauliflower rice, spinach and roasted red vegetables (R) • Oven-baked venison sausages (R) with garlic-roasted vegetables (R)

SNACKS	Fruit & Nuts/Seeds
If you tend to leave long gaps between meals, a small snack will help to maintain your energy levels and ensure that you arrive at the next meal hungry, rather than desperate. This will ensure you choose sustaining energy-boosting foods rather than grabbing a carby quick fix. Make sure every snack includes some form of protein!	• 1 apple, clementine, plum or other fruit with an edible skin PLUS 7–8 raw unsalted almonds, walnuts or hazelnuts or 1 tablespoon of pumpkin or sunflower seeds • 7–8 rosemary-roasted almonds (R) with an apple • A small pot of plain coconut or soya yoghurt with a tablespoon of fresh blueberries

DRINKS	Juice
Remember that just 2% dehydration can affect energy levels by up to 15%. Keeping yourself nicely topped up with fluid throughout the day in whichever form suits you best will definitely increase your Va Va Voom.	• Avoid pure fruit juices, especially anything in a carton, as these will send your blood sugar soaring. • Opt for freshly squeezed vegetable juices with just a small amount of fruit to sweeten it.

Fish	Vegetarian	Quick & Easy
• Salmon with lentils and garlic-roasted vegetables (R) • Prawn & pak choi stir fry (R) • Roasted haddock with citrus rice (R)	• Quinoa with garlic-roasted vegetables (R) • Vegetable & bean chilli with brown rice (R) • Lentil & vegetable casserole (R)	• 200g of low-sugar baked beans with grilled venison sausages

Oat or Rice Cakes	Vegetables	Cereal Bar or Ball
• 1–2 rough oatcakes or brown rice cakes with houmous, unsweetened nut butter or guacamole	• A handful of carrot, celery, pepper or cucumber sticks with 50g of houmous, or guacamole • Summer cup juice (R) • 15g of spicy roasted chickpeas (R)	Opt for something that contains plenty of nuts or seeds for a protein boost. Beware of sugary cereal bars, especially anything with large amounts of dried fruit (dates are commonly used to sweeten health bars and are very high in sugar).

Hot drinks	Water	Squash or cordial
• Herbal infusions such as peppermint, camomile, fennel or liquorice tea • Fruit teas • Rooibos/redbush tea (caffeine free) • Decaffeinated coffee	• Still and sparkling water • Coconut water (don't have more than 330ml per day because it can contain a lot of fruit sugar)	Where possible opt for low-sugar options. Try out interesting new flavours such as elderflower, ginger or raspberry. Added to sparkling water they make a lovely drink with a celebratory feel.

The Energiser Plan   The Super-Boost Plan

Days 8–10 – Cruising Days   Days 9–10 – Cruising Days

As you move into the last few days of the Va Va Voom plan, the Cruising Days are there to help you embed these energising food habits into your routine as you transition onto the Maintenance Plan. These days remain free from wheat, caffeine, alcohol, processed foods and refined sugar. They're also mostly dairy free, although natural yoghurt and cottage cheese are included again. You can also have limited amounts of rye bread or rye crispbread and brown rice, brown rice cakes or oatcakes.

CRUISING DAY GUIDELINES

- Remember to eat a combination of protein and fibre with every meal and snack
- Make sure you hit your vegetable-portion target with lunch and dinner
- Continue to eliminate wheat bread, pasta and couscous
- Enjoy either new potatoes or sweet potato maximum once a day
- Have a maximum of 2 slices of rye bread per day
- Choose either brown rice cakes or oatcakes or rye crispbread maximum once a day
- Reintroduce natural yoghurt, cottage cheese and goat's or sheep's milk and cheese; continue to avoid other forms of cow's milk; enjoy either goat's or sheep's cheese or cottage cheese maximum once a day
- Limit red meat to a maximum of twice a week; if you've already had it earlier in the programme, you may have used up your allowance already
- Eat at least 2 handfuls of cooked or raw leafy greens such as spinach, kale, cabbage, watercress and rocket per day
- Continue to eliminate alcohol, caffeine, wheat, refined sugar and processed foods

WHAT CAN I EAT ON A CRUISING DAY?

ENJOY (eat throughout the day)	LIMIT (follow the restrictions in the guidelines)	ELIMINATE
Beans	Brown rice, brown rice cakes	Alcohol
Chickpeas		Wheat bread and crackers, pasta, noodles, couscous
Dairy-free milk or yoghurt	Sweet fleshy fruit e.g. mango, pineapple, grapes	
Eggs	Goat's and sheep's cheese e.g. feta	Baked goods e.g. cakes, cookies, pastries, muffins, pies, tarts
Falafel	Cottage cheese	
Fruit with edible skin	New potatoes and sweet potato	
Houmous	Oats, rough oatcakes	Caffeine
Lentils	100% rye bread and rye crispbread	Chocolate, confectionery and crisps
Natural yoghurt	Lean red meat	
Nuts and nut butters	White meat	Cow's milk and cheese
Oily fish, white fish		Dried fruit
Quinoa		Ice cream
Seeds and seed butters		All other forms of potato e.g. fries, mashed or roast potato
Vegetables		Processed meat e.g. ham, salami, bacon
		Sugar and sugary foods

MEAL PLANNER FOR CRUISING DAYS

BREAKFAST	Eggs
A combination of protein- and fibre-rich foods is the best way to ensure sustained energy throughout the morning and to avoid cravings for energy-robbing foods. Choose one of these options or create your own breakfast, following the Va Va Voom protein–fibre principle.	• 1–2 scrambled or poached eggs with wilted spinach and fried mushrooms (use olive oil to scramble your eggs) • 1–2 scrambled, boiled or poached eggs with 1–2 slices of rye toast and dairy-free spread (use olive oil to scramble your eggs) • 1–2 poached eggs with mashed avocado on 1–2 slices of rye toast
LUNCH	Soup
Avoiding large portions of starchy carbohydrate at lunchtime will help to prevent the dreaded mid-afternoon slump. Baguette sandwiches, jacket potatoes or large portions of rice and pasta are likely to have you nodding off by 3pm! Remember to include plenty of protein with your lunch, as this will keep you going for longer.	• Lentil & tomato soup (R) with (optional) 2 rough oatcakes, 2 brown rice cakes or 1 slice of rye bread • Herby bean soup (R) with (optional) 2 rough oatcakes, 2 brown rice cakes or 1 slice of rye bread • Lemony chicken & vegetable soup (R) with (optional) 2 rough oatcakes, 2 brown rice cakes or 1 slice of rye bread

Grains	Fruit & Veg	Quick & Easy
• Overnight oats with dairy-free milk, fresh fruit and mixed seeds (R) • 40–50g of homemade granola (R) with natural yoghurt • Classic porridge with dairy-free milk, berries and chopped walnuts (R) • Quinoa porridge with dairy-free milk and fresh berries (R)	• Breakfast smoothie (R) • Pea power smoothie (R) • Vitality smoothie (R) • Fresh fruit salad with nuts and seeds (R) plus natural yoghurt	• 1–2 slices of rye toast with 50g of unsweetened peanut or almond butter

Salad	Hot Meal	Quick & Easy
Use the Va Va Voom Salad Bar on page 220 to help you construct your own salad e.g. • Quinoa & avocado salad (R) • Butternut squash & feta salad (R) • Smoked mackerel & beetroot salad (R)	• Jacket sweet potato with tuna mayo and spinach salad • Vegetable omelette (R) with rocket & pine nut salad • Courgette & pea frittata (R) with tomato & rocket salad	• Pre-cooked chicken breast or pre-poached salmon with ½ a bag of salad leaves, tomato and cucumber • Rye bread sandwich with chicken & salad, egg & salad or houmous & salad

DINNER	**Meat**
A careful combination of protein- and fibre-rich food will help to ensure blood sugar balance before bedtime, setting you up for a good night's sleep. Remember to follow the Va Va Voom Plate diagram to get the portions right.	• Shepherd's pie with crushed new potato topping (R) • Turkey meatballs with tomato sauce and brown rice (R) • Chicken & vegetable casserole (R) with new potatoes
SNACKS	**Fruit & Nuts/Seeds**
If you tend to leave very long gaps between meals, a small snack will help to maintain energy levels and ensure that you arrive at the next meal hungry, rather than desperate. This will ensure you choose sustaining energy-boosting foods rather than grabbing a carby quick fix. Make sure every snack includes some form of protein!	• 1 apple, clementine, plum or other fruit with an edible skin PLUS 7–8 raw unsalted almonds, walnuts or hazelnuts, or 1 tablespoon of pumpkin or sunflower seeds • 7–8 rosemary-roasted almonds (R) with an apple • A small pot of plain coconut or soya yoghurt with a tablespoon of fresh blueberries
DRINKS	**Juice**
Remember that just 2% dehydration can affect energy levels by up to 15%. Keeping yourself nicely topped up with fluid throughout the day in whichever form suits you best will definitely increase your Va Va Voom.	• Avoid pure fruit juices, especially anything in a carton, as these will send your blood sugar soaring. • Opt for freshly squeezed vegetable juices with just a small amount of fruit to sweeten it.

Fish	Vegetarian	Quick & Easy
• Grilled salmon with stir-fried vegetables and brown rice (R) • Prawn & pak choy stir fry (R) • Roasted haddock with citrus rice (R)	• Quinoa, courgette & goat's cheese-stuffed peppers (R) • Vegetable & bean chilli with brown rice (R) • Garlic-roasted vegetables with quinoa (R)	• Jacket sweet potato with dairy-free spread and low-sugar baked beans

Oat or Rice Cakes	Vegetables	Cereal Bar or Ball
• 1-2 rough oatcakes or brown rice cakes with houmous, unsweetened nut butter or soft goat's cheese	• A handful of carrot, celery, pepper or cucumber sticks with 50g of houmous, soft goat's cheese or guacamole • Spicy roasted chickpeas (R) • Pea power smoothie (R)	Opt for something that contains plenty of nuts and seeds for a protein boost. Beware of sugary cereal bars, especially anything with large amounts of dried fruit (dates, are commonly used to sweeten health bars and are very high in sugar).

Hot drinks	Water	Squash or cordial
• Herbal infusions such as peppermint, camomile, fennel or liquorice tea • Fruit teas • Rooibos/redbush tea (caffeine free) • Decaffeinated coffee	• Still and sparkling water • Coconut water (330ml maximum per day, as it can contain a lot of fruit sugar)	Where possible, opt for low-sugar options. Try out interesting new flavours such as elderflower, ginger or raspberry. Added to sparkling water they make a lovely drink with a celebratory feel.

THE WELLBEING WHEEL

Diet is just a part of the energy equation; it's important to think about lifestyle too. Managing your wellbeing is a crucial part of your Va Va Voom plan. A smart approach to sleep, exercise and relaxation will be fundamental to restoring your Va Va Voom.

Pick at least 2 options from the Exercise, Relaxation and Sleep sections of the Wellbeing Wheel and commit to them throughout the 10 days, logging them on the Wellbeing Tracker on the following pages.

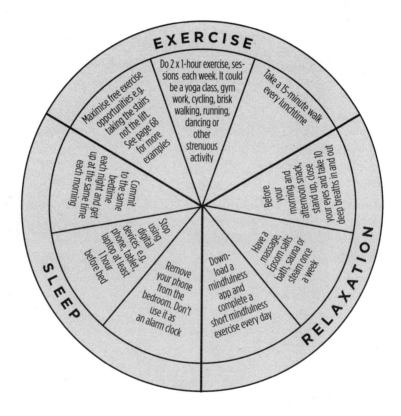

Wellbeing Tracker

	Example Day	Day 1	Day 2	Day 3	Day 4
EXERCISE	• 6pm spinning class. • Free exercise: walked to the next bus stop, instead of waiting at the usual one.				
RELAXATION	• 10.30am and 3pm – stepped away from my desk to do my 10 deep breaths. • 1pm – took a 15-minute walk in the park after lunch.				
SLEEP	• Used a radio alarm clock and left my phone charging in the kitchen overnight. • Put all digital devices away at 9pm, watched a film and went to bed.				

Day 5	Day 6	Day 7	Day 8	Day 9	Day 10

THE 10-DAY VA VA VOOM PLAN REVIEW

Now that you've completed your Va Va Voom plan, take a few minutes to think about any improvements you've experienced, what you've learned from the plan and which elements you'd like to permanently adopt into your lifestyle. You might want to do the Va Va Voom quiz again to track any improvement in your scores.

Which 3 things have you learned from the programme?
e.g. *a carb-heavy lunch makes me feel tired and lethargic* or *I sleep so much better when I don't drink alcohol.*

1.
2.
3.

Which 3 things will you carry on doing?
e.g. *take a packed lunch to work every day to make sure I have the type of lunch that suits me best* or *I'm going to carry on limiting the amount of alcohol I drink.*

1.
2.
3.

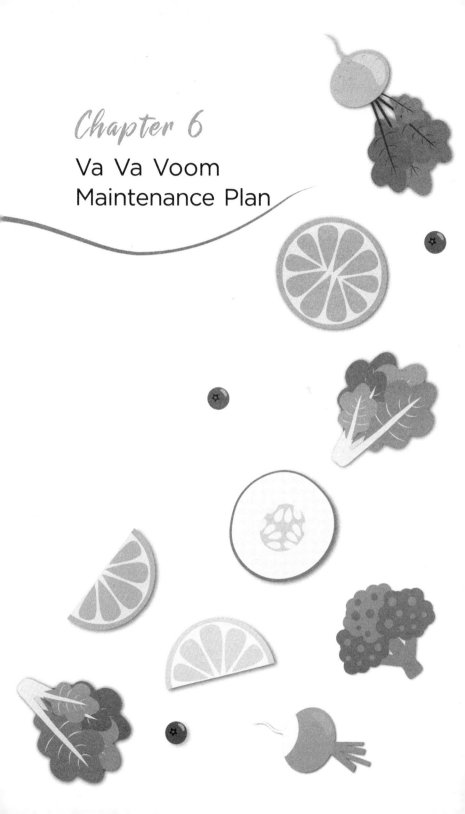

Chapter 6

Va Va Voom
Maintenance Plan

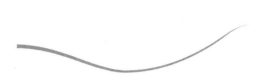

The Maintenance Plan is designed to help you continue to reap the benefits of your new-found energy by taking a flexible approach that is likely to be more sustainable and practical for you in the long term.

It provides a basic structure with specific advice around key potential energy-robbing areas. In order to achieve the most appropriate long-term plan for you, it's important to factor in your own personal learnings from the 10-day plan.

We are all biochemically individual and this means that each person will have had a different experience and will have discovered different potential triggers for their low energy as they progress through the Va Va Voom plan. Learning from your own personal experience and applying that to the Maintenance Plan will help you to create a sustainable diet and lifestyle which is specifically designed to support you and your energy levels in your daily life.

THE PRINCIPLES BEHIND THE MAINTENANCE PLAN

The 5 core principles of the Maintenance Plan are underpinned by the principles of the 10-Day Plan but they include more flexibility to help your new regime fit in with your schedule and to allow for social or business obligations.

1. Blood Sugar Balance

The blood sugar-balancing habits that you formed during the 10-day plan need to extend into the Maintenance Plan. This can be easily achieved by sticking to the core principles of blood sugar balance, even when you reintroduce some of the foods that had previously been eliminated. If you apply the following guidelines to your food choices, you won't go far wrong and you'll still have plenty of flexibility:

- make sure that every meal or snack contains protein in some form
- make a point of always choosing wholegrain foods such as wholemeal bread or brown rice
- don't fall back into the habit of skipping meals or leaving long gaps between meals
- limit your intake of caffeine and alcohol (see page 185) and avoid sugary foods

2. Reducing Inflammation

The 10-day plan was carefully structured to reduce underlying inflammation by eliminating certain pro-inflammatory food groups. The Maintenance Plan takes a more flexible approach that aims to be practical and sustainable, placing highly inflammatory foods firmly in the treat category, so that you can have them from time to time but aren't setting yourself up for a state of increased inflammation.

You'll see that wheat-based products such as bread, pasta and noodles now feature in their wholegrain forms. Wholewheat has a less inflammatory impact than refined wheat but, even so, it's advisable to remain within the Maintenance Plan guidelines of eating it maximum once a day. Dairy is now also included in the programme although milk and cheese, which can cause inflammation in sensitive individuals, should be limited to small amounts as set out in FAQ 8. Sugar, which is highly inflammatory, remains firmly in the 'Avoid' category and should be kept to an absolute minimum. Enjoying lots of anti-inflammatory foods such as oily fish, vegetables, nuts and seeds is a key principle of the plan.

3. Eat Plenty of Va Va Voom-Boosting Foods

It's highly important to keep including Va Va Voom-boosting foods in your diet and the 10-day plan should have instilled some positive new habits. The single most beneficial thing that you can do is prioritise vegetables in your diet because they are so rich in key nutrients for energy. Don't allow your vegetable portions to dwindle as you move on to the Maintenance Plan. Make sure that your fruit and veg intake is skewed in favour of vegetables, so that you're having 4 veg to 1 fruit portion or 5 veg to 2 fruit portions, for example. Sticking to the portion guidelines below for your main meals will ensure you consistently achieve 2 or 3 vegetable portions with each main meal.

The Va Va Voom Plate

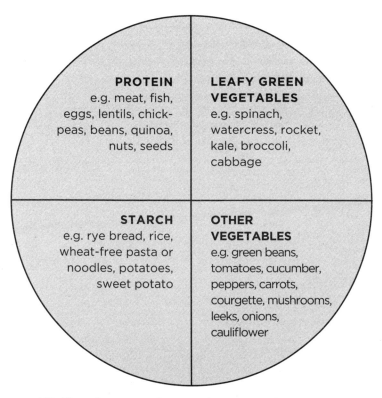

PROTEIN
e.g. meat, fish, eggs, lentils, chick-peas, beans, quinoa, nuts, seeds

LEAFY GREEN VEGETABLES
e.g. spinach, watercress, rocket, kale, broccoli, cabbage

STARCH
e.g. rye bread, rice, wheat-free pasta or noodles, potatoes, sweet potato

OTHER VEGETABLES
e.g. green beans, tomatoes, cucumber, peppers, carrots, courgette, mushrooms, leeks, onions, cauliflower

NB: if you're not eating starch at a meal, add another portion of vegetables, so that they represent 75% of the overall meal.

4. Avoid Va Va Voom-Robbing Foods

The Maintenance Plan is designed to allow flexibility around social occasions and to include the occasional treat, but Va Va Voom robbers such as sugar, alcohol and caffeine are all highly addictive. You'll need to treat these with caution to make sure that they don't sneakily become a daily habit which might undo all your good work during the 10-day plan.

5. The Wellbeing Wheels

Exercise, sleep and relaxation remain absolutely crucial to optimum energy as you move on to the Maintenance Plan. It's time to build on the wellbeing activities you introduced during the 10-day plan and make sure that they continue to form an integral part of your daily life on a weekly, monthly and quarterly basis. Review each Wellbeing Wheel so that you can consolidate the good habits you introduced over the 10 days and ensure they feature in your lifestyle in the long term.

HOW TO PREPARE FOR THE MAINTENANCE PLAN

The Maintenance Plan is more flexible than the 10-day plan to allow you to develop the most effective and personalised approach to boosting your Va Va Voom. This needs to be based on what you've learned from your experience following the 10-day plan.

Establish Your Goals

In order to establish your goals, you'll need to take some time to work out what you want them to be. These should be based on your review of the 10-day plan and the resolutions you formed at the end of the programme. You've probably identified certain elements of the plan that worked especially well for you; for example, you may have found that you slept better when you limited your caffeine intake or that eating bread makes you feel bloated and sluggish.

Using your learnings from the Va Va Voom Plan Review on page 169, set out your goals for the Maintenance Plan to help you keep your energy levels well on track. Create 4 Va Va Voom goals, including at least 1 wellbeing goal.

Your goals will need to be specific and measurable if you want to make them meaningful as this will help you track your progress, e.g. 'I will only have 1 cup of coffee a day'; 'I will only buy wholemeal bread' or 'I'm going to exercise 3 times a week' are more effective goals than 'I will try to drink less coffee' or 'I will eat more wholemeal bread' or 'I'm going to exercise regularly'. Setting out strategies to help you achieve your goals will make sure that each one is practical and sustainable.

If you know that you feel more energised and generally better after the 10-day plan but can't put your finger on which of the elements have directly affected you, which makes it hard to establish clear goals, you may wish to transition more slowly into the Maintenance Plan.

If you continue to follow the Cruising Day guidelines and reintroduce food or drink items individually and gradually over the next few weeks, you may be better able to identify the potential problem areas that affect your energy, sleep or overall wellbeing. You can then start to establish your goals for the Maintenance Plan.

My Va Va Voom Maintenance Goals

My Goal	How Will I Achieve It?
Example: I'm going to eat at least 4 portions of vegetables every day	• I'm going to make a vegetable smoothie at breakfast on weekend days • I'm going to have carrot sticks instead of fruit as my afternoon snack • I'm going to buy microwaveable packs of veg for dinner because they're quick and easy • I'm going to start making soup at home
1.	
2.	
3.	
4.	

WHAT CAN I EAT DURING THE MAINTENANCE PLAN?

Some of the foods that were eliminated in the 10-day plan can be reintroduced in small amounts in the Maintenance Plan. However, it's important not to undo all your good work by overdoing it, so pay particular attention to the Limit and Avoid lists and read the guidelines and the relevant FAQs to make sure you know exactly where you stand with the different foods and food groups.

ENJOY (eat throughout the day)	LIMIT (follow the restrictions in the guidelines)	AVOID (eat these as little as possible and never more than once a week)
Butter	Alcohol	Baked goods e.g.
Brown rice and	Caffeine	pies, pastries,
brown rice cakes	Wholegrain bread	sausage rolls
Cottage cheese	Cow's, goat's and	Processed meat
Eggs	sheep's milk	e.g. bacon, ham,
Fish	and cheese	salami
Fruit	Lean red meat	Ready meals and
White meat	Wholegrain pasta	convenience
Nuts	and noodles	foods e.g. pizza
Oats and oatcakes		Sweets, chocolate,
Pulses		confectionery
Quinoa		and crisps
Rye crispbread		Sugary foods
Seeds		
Vegetables		
Natural yoghurt		

THE MAINTENANCE PLAN FAQS

1. What do I do about caffeine?

Having eliminated caffeine from your diet for the past 10 days, this is a great opportunity to carry on with that or to at least reduce your consumption significantly, so that you're no longer reliant on it to keep you going throughout the day. If you're able to commit to little or no caffeine, it could have a big impact on the quality of your sleep and your energy levels.

2. How can I keep caffeine to a minimum?

- Limit yourself to a maximum of 200mg of caffeine per day e.g. 2 small coffees or 3 cups of tea
- Ask for 1 shot, instead of the standard 2 shots, when you're at a coffee shop
- Opt for a smaller cup size – a large coffee contains around 50mg more caffeine than a medium coffee and about 100mg more than a small coffee
- Don't brew your teabag for too long – leaving the bag in for 1-2 minutes instead of 4-5 minutes can halve the caffeine content
- Don't be fooled by green tea – it contains as much caffeine as black tea
- Don't overdo the cans of cola or energy drinks as these contain anything from 30 to 80mg of caffeine

CAFFEINE FACTS

- The maximum recommended dose for caffeine is 400mg per day
- A single espresso contains around 80mg of caffeine
- A small latte contains about 100mg of caffeine, a medium contains about 160mg and a large contains about 200mg
- Black or green tea contains 50-75g of caffeine, depending on brewing time
- Cola contains around 30mg per 330ml can
- Energy drinks contain around 80mg per 250ml can

3. Can I Drink Alcohol?

If you were in the habit of drinking even small amounts of alcohol on a regular basis, you'll have probably noticed a marked difference in the quality of your sleep and your energy levels when you eliminated it during your 10-day Va Va Voom plan.

While it's fine to enjoy a drink from time to time, it's important not to let alcohol creep back into your diet on a daily basis. A minimum of 3 consecutive alcohol-free days each week will make a big difference to the quality of your energy and your sleep. The consecutive element is important, because this allows your liver time to catch up with its many other important tasks, which include energy metabolism, instead of being constantly taken up with the business of detoxification.

4. How much alcohol can I drink?

Current UK guidelines are 14 units per week for both men and women. In the US, the guidelines advise a maximum of 12 units per week for women and 24 units for men.

5. What alcohol is best?

If you want to have plenty of Va Va Voom, it's best to keep the sugar content and alcohol units to a minimum when you're having a tipple, because this is a combination that can send your blood sugar soaring. Investing in a spirit measure and being aware of wine glass sizes for when you're serving drinks at home will help you keep track of what you're drinking.

When it comes to mixers, try to avoid sugary fizzy drinks, fruit juices or energy drinks; opt for low-sugar options such as soda water, sugar-free tonic water or sugar-free fizzy drinks.

Alcohol Facts

	Alcohol Units	Sugar Content
Red Wine (175ml)	2.3	0.3g
Medium White Wine (175ml)	2.3	5g
Rosé Wine (175ml)	2.3	6g
Sparkling Wine (125ml)	1.7	6g
Premium Lager (330ml)	3	8g
Bitter (1 pint)	2.3	12g
Spirits e.g. gin, vodka, whisky (25ml single measure)	1	Traces
Fortified Wine e.g. port, sherry (per 50ml measure)	1	5g

6. Can I eat bread?

You'll have noticed that bread was gradually phased out as you progressed through the plan. One reason for this was to help encourage you to increase the vegetable portions in your diet, as it's fairly common to over-rely on bread to bulk up a meal. The other reason is that the inflammatory nature of wheat can impact your energy levels, which is why some people find that large portions of wheat-based foods such as bread and pasta can make them feel sluggish and tired. This is a common issue if you tend to opt for refined white flour products, as these are especially inflammatory, as well as being low in fibre, which will affect your blood sugar levels.

Now you've moved on to the Maintenance programme, there's no reason not to reintroduce small amounts of bread or pasta into your diet, unless you've discovered that you feel better when you don't eat it at all.

7. What type of bread should I eat?

- Opt for wholegrain wheat or rye bread as this is rich in complex carbohydrate, which will help to maintain your blood sugar balance and support sustained energy levels.

It also tends to be less inflammatory than refined white bread.

- If you find that wheat bread makes you feel a bit bloated, try rye or even spelt, which is an ancient form of wheat that is usually less processed; some people find it easier to digest.

- Sourdough bread is another option which may make you feel less sluggish. Sourdough is made with a leaven that is derived from natural yeast and it can often be easier to digest than bread made with baker's yeast. The lengthy fermentation process that is used to develop the leaven may also help to stimulate the growth of beneficial bacteria in the gut.

- Gluten is a protein found in wheat, rye and barley and if you suspect that this is an issue for you it's advisable to consult your doctor to rule out coeliac disease. Coeliac disease is an autoimmune condition, one of the symptoms of which is gluten intolerance. Non-coeliac gluten intolerance is becoming increasingly recognised and you may find that keeping gluten to a minimum improves your energy levels. If so, opt for a gluten-free bread with minimal ingredients and avoid the more commercial options that contain multiple additives, preservatives and sugar.

8. Why do I have to limit some but not all dairy foods?

Milk and cheese feature in the 'Limited' category rather than the 'Enjoy' category because these are everyday foods that can easily creep into your diet in higher quantities than you realise and this may lead to an inflammatory response in some sensitive individuals. By limiting milk to 250ml per day, this will allow a sufficient amount for hot drinks, cereal or porridge, if this is your preference, but will ensure that it doesn't feature to excess. The same logic applies to cheese which is limited to a maximum of 3 portions per week in the Maintenance Plan guidelines. Natural yoghurt and cottage cheese usually feature in smaller quantities in the diet and have residual health benefits, which is why they can be enjoyed every day.

9. Why can I only eat fruit 3 times a day?

While fruit is generally very good for you and full of vitamins and minerals, it's worth remembering that it also contains plenty of fruit sugar. Eating large amounts of fruit can lead to a blood sugar spike, which will impact your energy levels in the long run. Placing the emphasis on vegetables rather than fruit will help to keep sugar levels to a minimum, provide plenty of fibre for sustained energy as well as lots of beneficial vitamins and minerals.

10. Can I eat dessert?

Most desserts are pretty sugary which means that they're always likely to impact your energy levels because of the effect on your blood sugar. 1–2 squares of dark chocolate would be a good low-sugar option, as would fresh fruit, as long as it doesn't make you bloated, which can sometimes happen if you eat it immediately after a meal. The best way to deal with dessert is to approach it as a treat – don't get into the habit of having a dessert with every meal and opt for a sweet herbal or a fruit tea instead. If you decide to treat yourself to a dessert, make sure it's worth it by waiting until a truly delicious option presents itself, rather than just having one automatically.

THE VA VA VOOM MAINTENANCE PLAN

MAINTENANCE PLAN GUIDELINES

- Make sure you continue to have a combination of protein and fibre with every meal and snack
- Avoid long gaps between meals
- Eat at least 2 handfuls of leafy greens such as spinach, watercress, rocket, cabbage and kale per day
- Limit your caffeine intake to a maximum of 200mg per day e.g. 2 small coffees or 3 teas
- If you're reintroducing alcohol, make sure you have at least 3 consecutive alcohol-free days each week
- Eat oily fish such as salmon, sardines or mackerel 3 times per week to boost anti-inflammatory omega 3 levels
- Aim for a maximum of 1 wheat-based meal per day so that it doesn't feature at each meal
- Limit milk to 250ml per day and have a portion of cheese no more than 3 times per week
- Aim for 5-7 portions of vegetables and fruit per day and skew the ratio in favour of vegetables e.g. 4 veg portions to 1 fruit portion or 5 veg portions to 2 fruit portions
- Limit your fruit intake to a maximum of 3 portions per day and choose a different fruit each time
- Limit red meat to a maximum of two portions per week
- Keep yourself well hydrated with 6-8 glasses of water per day. See Chapter 4 for advice on dehydration

MAINTENANCE MEAL PLANNER

This planner is designed to give you some guidance as you transition onto the Maintenance Plan. Anything that's flagged with the letter R will feature in the recipes in Chapter 7. It's fine to use your own

BREAKFAST	Eggs
Make sure you don't get complacent now that you've completed your initial plan. A protein-rich breakfast is still essential to supporting your energy levels throughout the morning, so don't slide back into your old habits.	• 2 flourless banana pancakes with blueberries (R) and natural yoghurt • 1–2 poached, scrambled or boiled eggs with 1–2 slices of wholemeal or rye toast (use olive oil to scramble your eggs) • 1–2 poached or scrambled eggs with wilted spinach, roasted tomatoes and fried mushrooms (use olive oil to scramble your eggs) • 1–2 poached eggs with ½ an avocado and 1–2 slices of sourdough toast
LUNCH	Soup
It's a good idea to vary your lunch and try lots of new things – you're more likely to stick to the Maintenance Plan in the long run if there's plenty of variety. If you get bored of your lunch you're more likely to be tempted by sugary or processed options that will disrupt your energy levels.	• Lentil & tomato soup (R) with a small wholemeal roll (optional) • Herby bean soup (R) with a small wholemeal roll (optional) • Lemony chicken & vegetable soup (R) with a small wholemeal roll (optional)

ideas and recipes of course, just make sure that your choice of
ingredients fits in with the Maintenance Plan guidelines.

Grains	Fruit & Veg	Quick & Easy
• 40–50g of homemade granola (R) with chopped kiwi fruit and natural yoghurt • Overnight oats with berries and seeds (R) • Classic porridge with berries and chopped walnuts (R) • Quinoa porridge with fresh berries (R)	• Overnight oats smoothie (R) • Pea power smoothie or juice (R) • Vitality smoothie (R) • Fresh fruit salad with nuts & seeds (R) and natural yoghurt	• Wholemeal bagel with smoked salmon and cream cheese • 50g of unsweetened peanut, cashew or almond butter on 1–2 slices of wholemeal or rye toast • 40–50g of low-sugar cereal, muesli or granola with a tablespoon of pumpkin and sunflower seeds and milk or dairy-free milk
Salad	**Hot Meal**	**Quick & Easy**
Use the Va Va Voom Salad Bar on page 220 to help you construct your own salad e.g. • Quinoa & avocado salad (R) • Prawn salad with brown rice and Asian dressing (R) • Smoked mackerel & beetroot salad (R) • Butternut squash & feta salad (R)	• Jacket sweet potato with tuna mayo and spinach salad • Grilled salmon with brown rice and stir-fried vegetables (R) • Courgette & pea frittata (R) with tomato & rocket salad	• Wholemeal or rye bread sandwich with protein e.g. chicken, tuna, egg or houmous PLUS at least 2 vegetables • Wholemeal pitta stuffed with falafel, houmous and mixed salad • A sushi box that includes mixed salad or edamame beans

DINNER	Meat
Keep up the good work at dinner time by ensuring that you're not overdoing the grains – if you've already had grains for breakfast, bread or pasta for lunch or you feel that you've had plenty of starch (e.g. bread, pasta, potatoes) throughout the day, then focus on vegetables and protein for dinner instead.	• Shepherd's pie with crushed new potato topping (R) • Turkey meatballs with tomato sauce and brown rice (R) • Oven-baked venison sausages with sweet potato mash and peas (R) • Grilled chicken with cauliflower rice, spinach and roasted red vegetables (R)
SNACKS	Fruit & Nuts/Seeds
Remember that you don't have to have a snack if you're not hungry, but it's important to avoid leaving long gaps between meals. If your blood sugar drops and your energy slumps, you're more likely to be tempted by energy robbers, which could undo all your good work.	• 1 apple, clementine, plum or other fruit with an edible skin PLUS 7–8 raw, unsalted almonds, walnuts or hazelnuts • 7–8 rosemary roasted nuts (R) with an apple
DRINKS	Juice
You've worked hard at keeping yourself hydrated during the 10-day plan, so don't let these good habits slide now. Remember that even mild dehydration can lead to a significant drop in energy levels, focus and concentration.	• Avoid pure fruit juices, especially anything in a carton as these will send your blood sugar soaring. • Opt for freshly squeezed vegetable juices with just a small amount of fruit to sweeten it.

Fish	Vegetarian	Quick & Easy
• Pan-fried salmon with green lentils and garlic-roasted vegetables (R) • Roasted haddock with citrus rice (R) • Sardine fishcakes (R) with root vegetable mash (R)	• Quinoa, courgette and goat's cheese-stuffed peppers (R) • Vegetable & bean chilli with brown rice (R) • Lentil & vegetable casserole • Vegetable omelette (R) with mixed salad	• Wholegrain pasta with tuna or cooked prawns and ½ a 350g jar of arrabbiata or puttanesca tomato sauce • Baked beans on wholemeal toast • Vegetable omelette (R) with goat's cheese and mixed salad

Oat or Rice Cakes	Vegetables	Cereal Bar or Ball
• 1–2 rough oatcakes or brown rice cakes with houmous, unsweetened nut butter or cottage cheese	• A handful of carrot, celery, pepper or cucumber sticks with 50g of houmous, soft goat's cheese or guacamole • 15g of spicy roasted chickpeas (R) • Tomato and carrot juice (R) with 7–8 raw nuts	Opt for something that contains plenty of nuts and seeds for a protein boost. Beware of sugary cereal bars, especially anything with large amounts of dried fruit (dates are commonly used to sweeten health bars and are very high in sugar).

Hot drinks	Water	Squash or cordial
• Herbal infusions such as peppermint, camomile, fennel or liquorice tea • Limited amounts of coffee, black tea or caffeinated health teas, such as matcha tea or green tea • Fruit teas • Rooibos/redbush tea (caffeine free) • Decaffeinated coffee	• Still and sparkling water • Coconut water (330ml per day maximum, as it can contain a lot of fruit sugar)	Where possible opt for low-sugar options. Try out interesting new flavours such as elderflower, ginger or raspberry. Added to sparkling water they make a lovely drink with a celebratory feel.

WELLBEING WHEEL

As with the 10-day plan, maintaining your Va Va Voom depends on managing your lifestyle as well as your diet. Establishing positive exercise, relaxation and sleep habits will make a significant difference to your energy levels. Using the 3 Wellbeing Wheels below, it's time to consolidate the wellbeing habits you established during the 10-day plan so that they become a natural part of your daily, weekly and quarterly schedules.

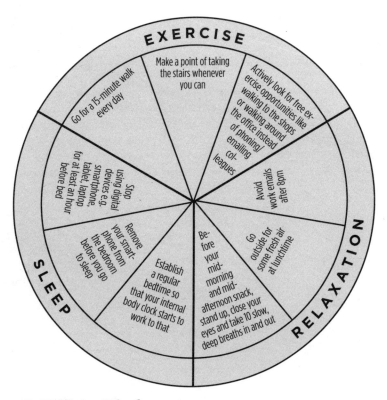

Daily Wellbeing Wheel

Choose two items from the Exercise, Sleep and Relaxation sections and commit to them on a daily basis so that they become natural habits.

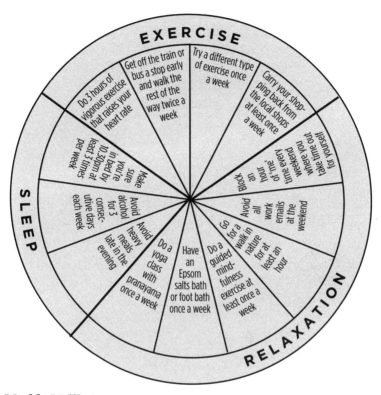

EXERCISE

Do 3 hours of vigorous exercise that raises your heart rate

Get off the train or bus a stop early and walk the rest of the way twice a week

Try a different type of exercise once a week

Carry your shopping back from the local shops at least once a week

Block an hour of 'me' time every weekend where you take time out for yourself

Avoid all work emails at the weekend

Go for a walk in nature for at least an hour

Do a guided mindfulness exercise at least once a week

Have an Epsom salts bath or foot bath once a week

Do a yoga class with pranayama once a week

Avoid heavy meals late in the evening

Avoid alcohol for 3 consecutive days each week

Make sure you're in bed by 10.30pm at least 3 times per week

SLEEP

RELAXATION

Weekly Wellbeing Wheel

Choose two items from the Exercise, Sleep and Relaxation sections
and schedule them into your diary for the week.

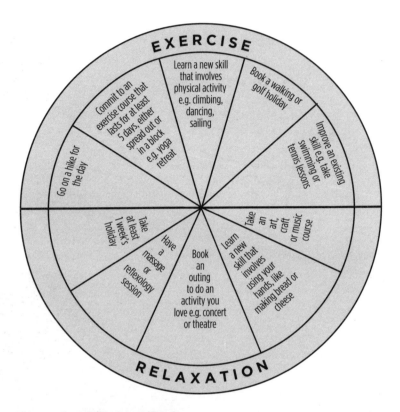

EXERCISE

Commit to an exercise course that lasts for at least 5 days, either spread out or in a block e.g. yoga retreat

Learn a new skill that involves physical activity e.g. climbing, dancing, sailing

Book a walking or golf holiday

Improve an existing skill e.g. take swimming or tennis lessons

Go on a hike for the day

Take at least 1 week's holiday

Have a massage or reflexology session

Book an outing to do an activity you love e.g. concert or theatre

Learn a new skill that involves using your hands, like making bread or cheese

Take an art, craft or music course

RELAXATION

Quarterly Wellbeing Wheel

Choose one item from the Exercise and Relaxation sections and schedule them into your diary once a quarter.

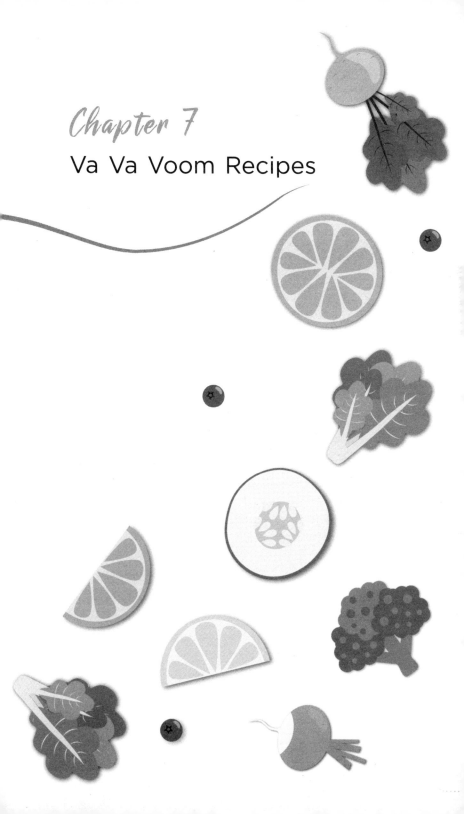

Chapter 7
Va Va Voom Recipes

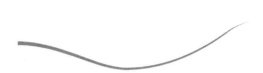

The Va Va Voom recipes provide a few examples of simple and practical meals, snacks and drinks, based around the principles of the 10-day Va Va Voom plan, that respect the guidelines for each phase to help you get started. Each recipe is flagged so that you know which phase of the 10-day plan it would be suitable for. All of these recipes can be used in the Va Va Voom Maintenance Plan.

It's absolutely fine to adapt your own favourite recipes or to try out something new if you like to be adventurous in the kitchen. You simply have to remember to check the ingredients and the portion guidelines for each phase of the programme.

For each recipe, you'll see a Va Va Voom factor that highlights a particular ingredient from each recipe, explaining why it can help you boost your energy levels so that you feel inspired to include it in your own recipes.

If you're not sure where to look for inspiration, here are some useful recipe websites which you might like to try:

- **www.bbcgoodfood.com:** my go-to website when I need inspiration. All the recipes are tested repeatedly so you know you can trust them to work every time. You can run a search of one or two ingredients for inspiration and then use the handy filters to fine-tune your search by cooking time and difficulty, type of meal and dietary restrictions.
- **www.foodsmatter.co.uk:** a very handy collection of free-from recipes which include meal recipes and baking recipes. Each recipe is coded so that you can easily pick out the ones that will suit your phase of the plan. For example, DF = dairy-free and WF = wheat-free.

- **www.nigelslater.com:** simple, practical and easy to use, any Nigel Slater recipe will be great, but he's a complete genius at making vegetables interesting, which will be a big help for reluctant vegetable eaters.
- **www.jamieoliver.com:** an extensive resource of very do-able healthy recipes with a brilliant search and filter function to help you stay within the Va Va Voom guidelines.
- **www.greatbritishchefs.com:** don't be put off by the name, you don't need to be a Cordon Bleu cook to manage these recipes; there are lots of great options for home cooks. This is another site where you can filter the recipes to suit your cooking ability, the time you have and the ingredients you want to work with.
- **www.allrecipes.co.uk:** a highly extensive collection of home-cooked recipes with a large free-from section.

There are also lots of great food and recipe blogs out there if you want to mix it up a bit. Try running a search on 'best food blogs' or type one or two key ingredients into a search engine and see which recipes and blogs come up.

Breakfast

Skipping breakfast won't help your Va Va Voom levels. If you normally have your evening meal at around 8pm and then wait until lunchtime to eat, this will leave your body without fuel for around 16 hours, which will have a direct impact on your energy, performance and concentration. If you've found that eating breakfast makes you feel hungry mid-morning so that you end up eating more, the chances are that your breakfast is low in protein. Sugary cereal, toast and jam or a fruit-based breakfast will all activate the insulin response as your body tries to process this blast of sugar. A protein-rich breakfast helps to buffer the impact of the sugar so that it's released more slowly into the bloodstream, providing a sustained level of energy.

These breakfast recipes provide some quick and easy examples of how to create a blood sugar-balancing breakfast by using a combination of protein and fibre. It's absolutely fine to adapt them if you prefer to use different fruits, nuts or seeds – just make sure you respect the relative proportions of the recipe, to keep your blood sugar on track.

FLOURLESS BANANA PANCAKES

Serves 2
Suitable for Intro, Booster
and Cruising Days

Ingredients

1 large banana

2 medium eggs

a dash of vanilla essence

1 tbsp rapeseed oil

1 tsp maple syrup

a handful of blueberries

a dollop of natural yoghurt (Intro and Cruising Days only)

Va Va Voom Factor

Eggs are one of the best sources of choline, a key player in supporting energy, concentration and memory.

Method

1. Peel and thoroughly mash the banana.

2. Beat in the eggs until the consistency is thick and fairly smooth and add a dash of vanilla essence.

3. Heat the oil in a non-stick frying pan.

4. Spoon about half the batter into the pan to make 2 pancakes and cook for 1–2 minutes on each side or until they're nicely browned; set aside on a plate to keep warm.

5. Repeat with the second half of the batter.

6. Serve with a teaspoon of maple syrup, a handful of blueberries and a dollop of natural yoghurt.

VEGETABLE OMELETTE

Serves 1
Suitable for Intro, Booster
and Cruising Days

Va Va Voom Factor
Egg yolk contains energy-boosting B vitamins and iron. It's also a good source of iodine, which supports healthy thyroid function.

Ingredients

1 tbsp rapeseed oil

your choice of 2 vegetables
   (e.g. a handful of sliced
   mushrooms; 1 shallot, finely sliced;
   a handful of cherry tomatoes; a handful of sliced green
   or red peppers; 2 handfuls of spinach leaves)

2–3 medium eggs, lightly beaten

25g goat's cheese (Intro and Cruising Days only)

salt and pepper

Method

1.   In a pan, heat the oil and gently fry your chosen vegetables until they're soft or the spinach is wilted. Remove from the pan and set aside on a warm plate.

2.   Season the eggs with salt and pepper and add them to the pan.

3.   Swirl the mixture around with a fork and lift the edges of the omelette with a spatula to encourage any uncooked egg towards the middle.

4.   When the egg is almost set, spoon the vegetable mixture into the middle and dot with the goat's cheese.

5.   Cook gently for another 1–2 minutes, or until the egg and cheese reaches your preferred texture.

6.   Fold the omelette in half over the vegetable mixture so that it's neatly wrapped, and serve.

HOMEMADE GRANOLA

Makes about 12 servings and keeps for up to 3 weeks in an airtight container.

Suitable for Intro, Booster and Cruising Days

Va Va Voom Factor
Sunflower seeds are packed with energy-boosting magnesium and zinc, which will give you a great start to the day.

Ingredients

2 tbsp maple syrup

4 tbsp rapeseed oil

200g rolled jumbo oats

75g pumpkin seeds

75g sunflower seeds

150g mixed nuts

Method

1. Preheat the oven to 170°C/150°C fan/gas mark 3. It's important to cook this on a low setting. If the oats are overdone they'll taste bitter, so feel free to adjust the settings according to your oven.

2. Pour the maple syrup into a pan with the oil and heat gently.

3. In a bowl, mix the oats and seeds together.

4. Pour the heated mixture into the bowl and mix together so the oats are evenly coated.

5. Spread the mixture out onto a baking tray.

6. Spread the mixed nuts out separately onto another baking tray.

7. Put them both in the oven for 21 minutes, turning the granola mixture 2 or 3 times.

8. Take them both out and move the granola around on the baking sheet with a spatula. As it cools down, it will harden and stick to the sheet unless you do this.

9. Chop the nuts roughly when they have cooled down, mix through the granola and store in an airtight jar ready for use.

OVERNIGHT OATS

Serves 1
Suitable for Intro, Booster
and Cruising Days

Ingredients

40g rolled oats

1 tbsp mixed sunflower and
   pumpkin seeds

1 tbsp mixed nuts, roughly
   chopped

½ small apple, peeled and grated

150ml unsweetened dairy-free milk

a handful of blueberries

**Va Va Voom
Factor**
Pumpkin seeds are
packed with protein,
magnesium and zinc.
They're also a great source
of copper, which is essential for energy production
and helps to support
iron absorption.

Method

1.   Measure out the oats into a cereal bowl.

2.   Stir in the seeds, chopped nuts and grated apple.

3.   Cover the mixture completely with the dairy-free milk.

4.   Leave in the fridge overnight to allow the liquid to be
     absorbed.

5.   Stir the blueberries through the mixture before
     serving.

CLASSIC PORRIDGE

Serves 1
Suitable for Intro, Booster and
Cruising Days

Ingredients

40g rolled oats

150ml unsweetened dairy-
   free milk

a handful of mixed frozen
   berries

1 tbsp walnuts, chopped

a dollop of natural yoghurt (Intro
   and Cruising Days only)

salt

Va Va Voom Factor
Walnuts are highly anti-inflammatory: not only are they an outstanding source of omega 3, they also contain antioxidant plant compounds, which help to reduce inflammation in the body.

Method

1. Put the oats into a saucepan and gently toast them over a low heat until they release a nutty fragrance, but be careful not to burn them.

2. Stir in the dairy-free milk and add a pinch of salt. Cook gently for about 5 minutes and keep stirring so that the mixture comes together smoothly as the oats start to absorb the milk. You can add more milk or water to adjust the consistency to suit you.

3. Add the berries for the last minute of cooking and heat through until they soften and start to stain the oats.

4. Serve topped with the walnuts and a dollop of natural yoghurt.

QUINOA PORRIDGE

Serves 1
Suitable for Intro, Booster
and Cruising Days

Ingredients

40g quinoa

50–100ml unsweetened dairy-
free milk

a handful of raspberries

a dash of vanilla essence and/or a
pinch of cinnamon

**Va
Va Voom
Factor**
Not only are raspber-
ries low in sugar, they also
contain plant compounds
which help to regulate the
breakdown of starch in
the body, maintaining
blood sugar
balance.

Method

1. Rinse the quinoa and add to 100ml of water in a saucepan.

2. Bring to the boil and then gently simmer for 10 minutes or until the grain starts to open up and the water is absorbed.

3. Stir in enough dairy-free milk to create your preferred consistency, add the raspberries and heat through for about 5 minutes.

4. Add a drop of vanilla extract and/or a pinch of cinnamon, to taste.

FRESH FRUIT SALAD

Serves 1
Suitable for Intro, Booster,
Cleansing and Cruising Days

Ingredients

½ apple, chopped (skin on)

a handful of blueberries

1 kiwi fruit, sliced

4 strawberries, halved

juice of ½ lemon

1 tbsp chopped nuts

1 tbsp mixed seeds

a dollop of natural yoghurt or dairy-free yoghurt (Intro, Booster and Cruising Days only)

Va Va Voom Factor
Kiwi fruit contains more vitamin C than an orange and it's a concentrated source of fibre, which helps to regulate blood sugar and promote sustained energy levels.

Method

1.   Prepare the fruit.

2.   Put the fruit into a bowl, add the lemon juice and stir thoroughly so that the fruit is covered.

3.   Sprinkle the nuts and seeds over the fruit and add a dollop of natural yoghurt or dairy-free yoghurt, depending on which phase of the programme you're in.

FRUIT AND VEG PLATTER

Serves 1
Suitable for Intro, Booster,
Cleansing and Cruising Days

Ingredients

½ avocado

1 carrot

1 small apple

1 kiwi fruit

1 slice of melon

6 cherry tomatoes, halved

½ lime

15g nuts, pumpkin seeds or sunflower seeds

Va Va Voom Factor

An avocado is a nutritional powerhouse, full of antioxidants, vitamins and minerals but also packed with anti-inflammatory monounsaturates, which support cognitive function, mental performance and mood.

Method

1. Peel and slice the avocado and cut the carrot into batons.

2. Cut the apple into quarters and slice thinly.

3. Peel and cut the kiwi fruit into thick slices.

4. Chop the melon into chunks.

5. Arrange everything on a platter, squeeze over the lime and sprinkle over the nuts or seeds before serving.

Smoothies and Juices

Homemade smoothies and juices are a perfect way to sneak lots of vegetables into your diet in one easy package; they easily mask the taste of vegetables that you know are good for you but perhaps you're not so keen on eating!

To make sure that your smoothies and juices have the Va Va Voom factor, it's important to steer clear of highly fruity mixes because these will give you a powerful blast of sugar, sending your blood sugar soaring and disrupting your energy levels. Small bottles of fruit smoothies, such as mango and pineapple or blueberry and banana, from grab-and-go outlets can contain the equivalent of 7–8 teaspoons of sugar.

The Va Va Voom smoothies and juices contain limited fruit and a combination of vegetables, oats, nuts or seeds to give you the best possible start to the day with plenty of vitamins, minerals and fibre. Once you feel comfortable, you can try making your own concoctions; here are a few tips to get you started:

- Every smoothie needs a base to give it that creamy texture: banana, nut butter, oats, natural yoghurt or avocado all work well.
- Choose your liquid: this will probably be a dairy-free milk, filtered water or coconut water. You'll only need a small amount.
- Pick your fruit and vegetables carefully. The strength of your blender will play a part here, so opt for easily blended veg such as spinach or other leafy greens, herbs and soft fruit such as berries or roughly chopped apple, pear or mango.

- Feel free to adjust the consistency of your smoothies by adding water or ice. If you prefer a thick and creamy texture, try using frozen fruit – it's a good way of creating a chilled smoothie without watering it down.
- Feel free to add a little flavouring, such as a pinch of cinnamon or a dash of vanilla essence.
- If you're juicing, you can add pretty much any combination that works for you, although it's important to keep fruit to a minimum and ramp up the vegetables. Using starchy vegetables such as carrot or beetroot will add some natural sweetness if a pure green juice is too much for you. Adding a lemon can also help neutralise the bitterness of green vegetables.
- If you've got the time and don't mind the extra washing up, a combination of juicing and blending can produce a lovely drink with a smoother consistency. This allows you to juice some tougher fruit and vegetables without having to peel and chop them and then you can add in some more delicate options to the blender, such as avocado, banana, nut butter or herbs.

VITALITY SMOOTHIE

Serves 1
Suitable for Intro, Booster and
Cruising Days

Ingredients

100ml unsweetened dairy-
   free milk

½ avocado, roughly
   chopped

1 banana, roughly chopped

a handful of parsley

2 large handfuls of spinach

**Va Va Voom
Factor**
Parsley is absolutely
packed with vitamins C
and K, both essential for
the citric acid cycle phase
of energy production. It's
also a good source of
B vitamins and iron.

Method

1.   Put the milk into the blender first and then add the
      avocado and banana, pulsing a few times to break it
      down.

2.   Add the parsley and spinach and blend until the
      mixture is smooth and creamy.

OVERNIGHT OATS SMOOTHIE

Serves 1
Suitable for Intro, Booster and
Cruising Days

Ingredients

30g rolled oats

1 apple, grated

1 tbsp pumpkin or sunflower
   seeds

200ml unsweetened dairy-free milk

½ banana, roughly chopped

a pinch of cinnamon

**Va Va Voom
Factor**
Soaking your oats over-
night will make them
more digestible and will
reduce the level of phytic
acid which inhibits the
absorption of iron.

Method

1. Put the oats, apple and seeds into a bowl and cover
    with dairy-free milk. You need about double the
    amount of milk to oats. Leave in the fridge overnight.

2. Remove the oat mixture from the fridge and put into
    the blender with another 50ml of dairy-free milk.

3. Add the banana and blend until the mixture is
    smooth.

4. Serve with a dusting of cinnamon on top.

GORGEOUS GREEN JUICE OR SMOOTHIE

Serves 1
Suitable for Intro, Booster,
Cleansing and Cruising Days

Ingredients

1 apple, chopped

½ cucumber,
   roughly chopped

a handful of basil leaves

juice of ½ lime

½ avocado, sliced

> **Va Va Voom Factor**
> Cucumbers are a bit of a one-stop energy shop. They're high in vitamin K and also contain vitamin C, B vitamins, copper and magnesium – all essential components of the citric acid cycle.

Smoothie Method

1. Core the apple and add to the blender with the cucumber and pulse the mixture until it starts to break down.

2. Add the basil, lime juice and avocado and blend until smooth. Adjust the consistency with water to suit your preference. Depending on how powerful your blender is, it can be quite a thick consistency; you may prefer it as a juice.

Juice Method

1. Juice the apple and the cucumber and pour the mixture into your blender.

2. Add the basil, lime juice and avocado and blend thoroughly. This creates a perfect creamy consistency – as long as you don't mind the extra washing up.

PEA POWER SMOOTHIE

Serves 1
Suitable for Intro, Booster,
Cleansing and Cruising Days

Va Va Voom Factor

Peas are a natural blood sugar balancer, containing an ideal combination of protein and fibre to keep you going for longer. They're also an excellent source of energy-boosting B vitamins, zinc, vitamin C and iron.

Ingredients

2 handfuls of frozen green peas

1 apple, cored and roughly chopped

¼ cucumber, roughly chopped

½ avocado, sliced

2 handfuls of baby spinach

2–3 mint leaves

Method

1. Add the peas to the blender and pulse to break down the ice.

2. Add the apple and cucumber with about 100ml of filtered water and pulse until they start to form a mixture.

3. Add the avocado, spinach and mint and blend until smooth. You may need to add another 50ml of water if the mixture is too thick.

4. This is another smoothie where you can get a more uniform texture by juicing the apple and cucumber first and then adding them to the rest of the ingredients for blending.

BREAKFAST SMOOTHIE

Serves 1
Suitable for Intro, Booster and
Cruising Days

Va Va Voom Factor
Cashews are full of copper which we need for the production of red blood cells that provide the oxygen we need to produce energy.

Ingredients

30g rolled oats

1 tbsp sunflower seeds

250ml unsweetened dairy-free milk

a handful of frozen mixed berries

½ banana, roughly chopped

25g unsweetened cashew butter (or other preferred nut butter)

Method

1. Measure out the oats and sunflower seeds into a bowl and cover with dairy-free milk. You need to use about twice the amount of milk to oats. Leave in the fridge to soak overnight.

2. In the morning, add the berries to the blender and pulse until the ice is broken down.

3. Add the oat mixture, banana and about 100ml of dairy-free milk and start to blend the mixture.

4. Add the cashew butter gradually through the feeder at the top of the blender so that it doesn't clog up the blades and then blend the whole mixture thoroughly before serving.

SUMMER CUP JUICE

Serves 1
Suitable for Intro, Booster,
Cleansing and Cruising Days

Va Va Voom Factor

Anti-inflammatory kale contains large amounts of sulphur compounds which help to reduce the toxic load in the liver that can make us feel sluggish.

Ingredients

a handful of kale

½ cucumber

½ sweetheart cabbage

a handful of mint leaves

1 large apple

4–5 strawberries

Method

1. Feed all the ingredients into your juicer, juice and serve.

2. If you want a stronger mint flavour, hold back the mint and strawberries and juice the other ingredients first. Then add the juice to your blender with the mint leaves and strawberries and blend thoroughly.

BOOSTER JUICE

Serves 1
Suitable for Intro, Booster,
Cleansing and Cruising Days

Ingredients

1 medium courgette

½ cucumber

1 large apple

Va Va Voom Factor
Polyphenols found in apples help to prevent blood sugar spikes by slowing down the rate of glucose absorption, providing a more sustained source of energy.

Method

Feed the ingredients through your juicer and serve.

TOMATO AND CARROT JUICE

Serves 1
Suitable for Intro, Booster,
Cleansing and Cruising Days

Ingredients

3 large tomatoes

1 carrot

Va Va Voom Factor

Carrots are a great all-round source of vitamins B1, B3, B5, folate, copper and vitamin C, all of which are essential for the body's energy-production process.

Method

1. Chop the tomatoes in half and pass through the juicer with the carrot.

2. This is a delicious fresh juice if you use really good-quality tomatoes, but you can always spice it up by blending it with a teaspoon of chopped onion and a few parsley leaves, if need be.

CARROT AND APPLE JUICE

Serves 1
Suitable for Intro, Booster,
Cleansing and Cruising Days

Va Va Voom Factor
Regular consumption of apples may help to improve the balance of beneficial bacteria in the gut, enhancing the absorption of energy-boosting nutrients.

Ingredients

a thumbnail-sized piece of
  ginger

1 large apple

3 large carrots

Method

1. Peel and quarter the ginger.

2. Halve the apples and add to your juicer with the ginger and the carrots.

Lunch

It's crucial to get lunch right if you want to improve your energy and performance for the rest of the day. If the mid-afternoon energy slump is a familiar scenario for you, it's time to take a serious look at what you're having for lunch.

Blood sugar balance is a key factor here, so make sure that your lunch contains plenty of protein – protein-rich foods such as meat, fish, eggs and quinoa will help to slow down the release of carbohydrate in the body, which will keep you going for longer. Steer clear of refined or simple carbohydrates such as a hefty baguette sandwich, huge portions of white rice or a massive jacket potato, as these will lead to a blood sugar crash that could have you nodding off during a crucial meeting in the afternoon.

Focusing on fibre-rich options such as vegetables and wholegrains like rye bread or brown rice will keep your blood sugar nice and stable, your energy levels steady and your brain firing on all cylinders. Some people may find that even with wholegrain starch, too much makes them feel sluggish in the afternoon, and if you're one of them, keep your carbohydrate portion small and boost up the meal with vegetables and protein.

VA VA VOOM SALAD BAR

If you don't have the time to come up with new and inspiring salads, the Va Va Voom Salad Bar will make it easy for you. Follow the instructions from each column to help you make a balanced salad. Each section should amount to 25% of the salad, so make sure you manage your portions carefully. And don't forget to select the ingredients that are relevant for the phase of the programme that you're currently working on.

1. PICK YOUR INGREDIENTS

Choose 1 base and add a fist-sized portion	Add 2 handfuls of leafy greens	Pick at least 2 vegetables	Top with at least 1 protein source, a fist-sized portion
Brown rice	Spinach	Mushrooms	Egg
Quinoa	Lamb's	Tomatoes	Chicken
Wholegrain	lettuce	Peppers	Turkey
pasta	Kale	Broccoli	Salmon
Beetroot	Watercress	Green beans	Tuna
Sweet potato	Rocket	Celery	Sardines
Pumpkin	Cabbage	Grated carrot	Smoked
Butternut	Mixed leaves	Cucumber	mackerel
squash	Fresh lettuce	Mangetout	Goat's
Beans e.g.		Sugar snap	cheese
kidney,		peas	Feta
borlotti,		Avocado	Nuts
fava		Artichoke	Seeds
Lentils		hearts	Tofu
Chickpeas		Grated	
		courgette	
		Beansprouts	
		Chicory	
		Fennel	

2. SPICE IT UP!

If you find salads a bit dull, there are lots of things you can do to add flavour. Pick one herb and roughly chop or tear the leaves and then mix it in with your leafy greens. It'll transform your lettuce! If you like stronger flavours, choose something from the Zing column – don't overdo it though or your salad might become a bit overpowering.

Fresh herbs	Zing
Basil	Grated onion
Mint	Crushed garlic
Parsley	Chilli flakes
Coriander	Shaved ginger
Sage	Chopped olives
Thyme	Sundried tomatoes
Oregano	Jalapeño peppers
	Gherkins
	Pomegranate seeds
	Fresh figs

3. ADD YOUR DRESSING

These quantities make an individual portion but it's fine to increase them if you're making a salad to share or would like to store it in a jar for another day. Dressing should keep for up to a week in the fridge. Don't forget to mix it up again if it's been standing for a while as the ingredients may separate. Using olive oil with infused lemon, orange, garlic, chilli or herbs is a great way to add extra flavour to your dressing.

French dressing	Yoghurt dressing
1 tbsp extra virgin olive oil; 2 tsp red wine vinegar; 1 tsp Dijon mustard. Season with pepper and mix well.	1 tbsp natural yoghurt; juice of ½ small lemon; 2 tsp finely chopped parsley or mint. Season with pepper and mix well.
Asian dressing	**Spicy salsa**
1 tbsp sesame oil; 1 tsp soy or tamari soy sauce; 1 tsp lemon juice; ½ tsp finely minced ginger; ½ tsp crushed garlic. Season with pepper and mix well.	5 cherry tomatoes, quartered; ½ small red onion, chopped; 1 garlic clove, crushed; 1 red chilli, deseeded and roughly chopped; a handful of coriander; juice of 1 small lime. Add everything to a blender and pulse to make a rough purée. Season to taste.

Over the next few pages are a few example salads to get you started.

SMOKED MACKEREL AND BEETROOT SALAD

Serves 1
Suitable for Intro, Booster and Cruising Days

Ingredients

1 fillet hot-smoked mackerel

3 baby beetroot, cooked

80g raw broccoli florets

2 handfuls of watercress

6 cherry tomatoes, halved

French dressing (see page 222)

Va Va Voom Factor

Anti-inflammatory beetroot supports detoxification, reducing the load on the liver that can impact on our energy. Recent studies have shown that beetroot juice enhances endurance and performance in athletes.

Method

1. Use a fork to flake the mackerel into small pieces.
2. Cut the beetroot into quarters.
3. Split the broccoli into small, bite-sized florets.
4. Mix all the ingredients together and toss with the French dressing.

QUINOA AND AVOCADO SALAD

Serves 1
Suitable for Intro and
Cruising Days

Va Va Voom Factor

They may be small but beansprouts contain many of the catalyst vitamins and minerals we need to activate the citric acid cycle and are especially high in vitamins C and K.

Ingredients

120g quinoa

500ml vegetable stock

½ avocado, cut into small chunks

¼ cucumber, diced

80g beansprouts

2 handfuls of mixed leaves

1 tomato, sliced

a pinch of chilli flakes

Mint yoghurt dressing (see page 222)

Method

1. Put the quinoa and the stock into a pan and bring to the boil. Cook for 12–15 minutes until the quinoa has softened and opened up.

2. Rinse the cooked quinoa with cold water and leave to drain until dry.

3. Put all the ingredients into a salad bowl, spoon over the yoghurt dressing and toss it through the salad.

BUTTERNUT SQUASH AND FETA SALAD

Serves 2
Suitable for Intro and
Cruising Days

Va Va Voom Factor
Spinach is a top source of magnesium, iron and a whole range of B vitamins, so eating plenty of it will keep your energy-production process in fine working order.

Ingredients

1 tsp lemon-infused olive oil

500g butternut squash, peeled and cut into 2.5cm cubes

4 handfuls of baby spinach leaves

10 cherry tomatoes, halved

¼ cucumber, diced

1 x 400g tin of Puy lentils, rinsed and drained

French dressing (see page 222)

25g feta cheese

a handful of chopped parsley

Method

1. Preheat the oven to 200°C/180°C fan/gas mark 6.

2. Drizzle the lemon olive oil over the butternut squash cubes, making sure they're thoroughly coated.

3. Place on a baking sheet and roast for about 25 minutes until they're cooked through, turning occasionally.

4. Place the spinach, tomatoes, cucumber and lentils in a salad bowl and toss with the French dressing.

5. Top with the roasted butternut squash, crumble over the feta and sprinkle with the chopped parsley.

MIXED VEGETABLE SALAD WITH SPICY SALSA

Serves 1
Suitable for Intro, Booster,
Cleansing and Cruising Days

Ingredients

1 chicory

2 large handfuls of
   watercress

a handful of raw broccoli florets

1 carrot, grated

3 chestnut mushrooms, finely sliced

¼ cucumber, diced

Spicy salsa (see page 222)

Va Va Voom Factor

Chicory is especially high in folate and choline, which are two critical catalyst nutrients in the energy-production process. It's also an excellent source of fibre, providing sustained energy levels.

Method

1. Cut the woody end off the chicory, slice in half lengthways and cut out the core. Slice the leaves crossways and place in a salad bowl.

2. Add all the other vegetables, toss thoroughly with the spicy salsa and serve.

PRAWN SALAD WITH BROWN RICE

Serves 1
Suitable for Intro, Booster and
Cruising Days

Ingredients

75g cooked king prawns

1 tbsp Asian dressing (see
  page 222)

2 large handfuls of baby spinach
  leaves

8 cherry tomatoes, halved

1 spring onion, sliced diagonally

¼ cucumber, diced

75g pre-cooked brown rice

**Va
Va Voom
Factor**
Super high in fibre
which keeps your blood
sugar nicely balanced,
brown rice is also packed
with selenium which
keeps your thyroid in
good working
order.

Method

1.   In a salad bowl, marinate the prawns in the Asian
      dressing for at least an hour and then remove them
      with a slotted spoon.

2.   Add all the vegetables and the rice to the dressing
      and toss thoroughly so that everything is well coated.

3.   Scatter over the prawns and serve.

SPICY GREEN AND RED SALAD

Serves 1
Suitable for Intro, Booster,
Cleansing and Cruising Days

Ingredients

2 handfuls of baby spinach

3 mushrooms, finely sliced

½ avocado, diced

100g courgette, grated

6 cherry tomatoes, halved

½ red pepper, sliced

Spicy salsa (see page 222)

15g pine nuts

Va Va Voom Factor

Nutritious mushrooms are full of energy-boosting B vitamins, folate and choline. They have anti-inflammatory properties and are a great source of copper, which we need to oxygenate our body, and selenium, which is vital for thyroid function.

Method

1. Add all the vegetables to a salad bowl and toss with the salsa.

2. Sprinkle with the pine nuts and serve.

HERBY BEAN SOUP

Serves 4
Suitable for Intro, Booster and
Cruising Days

Ingredients

1 tbsp rapeseed oil

1 carrot, chopped

1 onion, chopped

1 x 400g tin of borlotti beans

1 x 400g tin of butter beans

750ml vegetable stock

a few sprigs of thyme and rosemary

15g pine nuts

Va Va Voom Factor

Beans contain a combination of protein and fibre in one easy package, making them a perfect blood sugar-balancing option. They're also a great plant source of iron.

Method

1. Heat the oil in a saucepan and gently cook the vege-tables for about 10 minutes until they are soft and the onions transparent.

2. Add the beans and the stock, with a few sprigs of thyme and rosemary.

3. Simmer for at least 20 minutes to allow the flavours to infuse and then remove the herbs.

4. Pour the mixture into a blender, or use a hand blender for a more rustic, chunky effect.

5. Gently dry-fry the pine nuts to toast them.

6. Serve with a drizzle of olive oil and garnish with the pine nuts.

TOMATO AND BASIL SOUP

Serves 2
Suitable for Intro, Booster,
Cleansing and Cruising Days

Va Va Voom Factor
Tomatoes are outstandingly rich in antioxidants, especially lycopene which has anti-inflammatory properties and supports blood flow, ensuring that the oxygen we need for energy is delivered to all our muscles, cells and tissues.

Ingredients

1 tbsp rapeseed oil

1 onion, finely chopped

1 garlic clove, crushed

5 large tomatoes

3 sun-dried tomatoes

500ml vegetable stock

2 handfuls of basil leaves

salt and pepper

Method

1. Heat the oil in a saucepan, add the onions and cook over a low heat until they are soft and transparent but not brown.

2. Add the garlic and gently cook through for about a minute.

3. Roughly chop the fresh tomatoes and add them to the pan with the sun-dried tomatoes, vegetable stock and a pinch of salt and pepper.

4. Bring to the boil. Turn down the heat and simmer for about 20 minutes.

5. Roughly tear the basil leaves and stir through the soup before taking it off the heat.

6. Add to your blender and blitz until smooth.

BROCCOLI AND SAGE SOUP

Serves 2
Suitable for Intro, Booster,
Cleansing and Cruising Days

Ingredients

1 tbsp olive oil

1 medium carrot, sliced

1 small onion, diced

1 celery stick, sliced

a head of broccoli (about
　300g)

1 tbsp finely chopped chives

1 tbsp sage leaves

1 litre vegetable stock

salt and pepper

Va Va Voom Factor

Protective plant compounds in broccoli help to reduce inflammation and the level of toxins in the body which might be robbing you of energy. Broccoli is packed with the B vitamins, vitamin C, copper, zinc and magnesium we need to produce energy.

Method

1.　Heat the oil in a saucepan and add the carrot, onion and celery. Cover and sweat the vegetables over a low heat for 5–10 minutes until soft but not brown.

2.　Roughly chop the broccoli and add to the pan with the chives, sage and vegetable stock.

3.　Season with salt and pepper and bring to the boil. Turn down the heat and simmer for 8–10 minutes until the broccoli is just soft. Don't cook for too long or you'll lose the lovely green colour.

4.　Add to your blender and blitz until smooth.

LENTIL AND TOMATO SOUP

Serves 4
Suitable for Intro, Booster
and Cruising Days

Va Va Voom
Factor
Packed with protein and
fibre, lentils will balance
your blood sugar in one
quick fix. They are also a
great plant source of
iron.

Ingredients

1 tbsp olive oil

1 tsp cumin seeds

1 medium leek, finely sliced

1 celery stick, sliced

1 carrot, sliced

6 large tomatoes

1 litre vegetable stock

180g red lentils

salt and pepper

Method

1. Heat the oil in a large saucepan and gently fry the
    cumin seeds until they release their flavour.

2. Add the leek, celery and carrot. Cover the pan and
    sweat the vegetables over a low heat until they are soft.

3. Roughly chop the tomatoes and add them to the pan
    with the stock.

4. Cook gently for about 5 minutes until the tomatoes
    start to soften and then add the lentils.

5. Season with salt and pepper, bring to the boil and
    then simmer over a low heat for about 20 minutes
    until the lentils are soft.

6. Add to your blender and blitz until smooth. Add some
    water if you prefer a thinner consistency.

LEMONY CHICKEN AND VEGETABLE SOUP

Serves 6
Suitable for Intro, Booster
and Cruising Days

Va Va Voom Factor
Celery is highly anti-inflammatory and packed with antioxidants. It's also a great source of folate and may help to reduce blood pressure.

Ingredients

1 whole chicken (about 1kg)

4 onions, thinly sliced

6 carrots, thickly sliced

6 celery sticks, thickly sliced

3 garlic cloves

a few sprigs of lemon thyme

zest and juice of 1 lemon

salt

Method

1. Cut the chicken into 4–5 pieces and place them in a pot. Cover with water, add a teaspoon of salt and bring to the boil.

2. Skim the foam off the top and add the onions, carrots, celery, garlic and thyme.

3. Cover and simmer for about 30 minutes. Remove the chicken breast so that it doesn't overcook and go dry.

4. Shred the chicken breast, toss with the lemon zest and half the lemon juice and set aside.

5. Add the rest of the lemon juice to the pot and cook for another 35–40 minutes until the meat is tender and falling away from the bone.

6. Remove the rest of the chicken and the thyme sprigs from the pot. Pull the meat from the bone.

7. Add all the chicken back to the pot with the vegetables and warm through for about 5 minutes before serving.

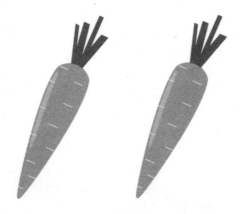

COURGETTE AND PEA FRITTATA

Serves 4
Suitable for Intro and
Cruising Days

Ingredients

1 tbsp olive oil

1 small onion, finely sliced

1 garlic clove, crushed

140g fresh or fully defrosted
   peas

1 large courgette, grated

6 eggs

a handful of finely chopped
   mint leaves

75g feta

**Va Va Voom
Factor**
Peas contain
antioxidant and
anti-inflammatory
compounds which
support cardiovascular
health, promoting the flow
of blood and oxygen
around the body, which
is essential for gener-
ating energy.

Method

1. Preheat the grill to high.

2. Heat the oil in a non-stick, grill-safe frying pan and
    gently fry the onions until they are soft and
    transparent.

3. Add the garlic, peas and courgette, cover and cook
    over a low heat for about 5 minutes until the mixture
    has reduced down and the vegetables are soft but
    not brown.

4. In the meantime, beat the eggs and stir the mint
    through them.

5. Break the feta into small cubes and add to the egg,
    stirring carefully so the cubes don't break up.

6. When the vegetable mix is ready, pour in the egg and move the vegetables around with a wooden spatula, so that the egg is evenly distributed though the mixture.

7. Cook over a low heat for 5 minutes, or until the mixture is almost set.

8. Put the pan under the grill for 3–4 minutes or until the frittata is golden and set.

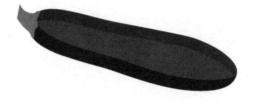

Dinner

The evening meal is often the time when things can go a bit wrong and over-indulgence creeps in as you relax after a busy day. If you've been following the plan carefully and sticking to the guidelines about meal portions and timing, you're far less likely to give in to temptation.

The important thing here is to plan your meals in advance and make sure that you have all the ingredients you need. Remember how important vegetables are to your Va Va Voom and make sure that they add up to at least 50% of the overall meal – you'll need to be having 2 or 3 portions of different vegetables to hit that target. Don't feel obliged to have the starch portion if you wouldn't normally eat rice, potatoes, pasta or bread in the evening; you can simply increase the overall vegetable portion to 75% of the meal.

Blood sugar balance remains an essential factor here – a balanced evening meal of protein and fibre will keep your blood sugar nice and stable so that your stress hormones aren't activated during the night and you can have a refreshing night's sleep.

These simple recipes provide a few examples to get you started. Feel free to swap the ingredients around to suit your taste or to use your own preferred recipes. All you need to do is stick to the ingredient and portion guidelines for each phase of the plan and you'll be well on track.

TURKEY MEATBALLS WITH TOMATO SAUCE

Makes 15 meatballs (4–5 meatballs per serving)
Suitable for Intro, Booster and Cruising Days

Ingredients

300g turkey breast mince

½ onion, finely chopped

1 large garlic clove, crushed

1 tsp garam masala

1 tsp cumin

½ tsp cayenne pepper

1 tbsp finely chopped coriander

1 egg, beaten

30g gluten-free fresh breadcrumbs

1 tbsp rapeseed oil

125g pre-cooked brown rice

Tomato sauce (see page 240)

salt and pepper

Va Va Voom Factor

As well as being packed with lean protein, turkey is an excellent source of all the B vitamins required for the chain reaction of energy production.

Method

1.   Preheat the oven to 180°C/160°C fan/gas mark 4.

2.   Put the mince, onion and garlic into a mixing bowl.

3.   Add the garam masala, cumin and cayenne, plus a pinch of salt and pepper and mix thoroughly together so that there's an even distribution of each ingredient. Then stir in the chopped coriander.

4.   Pour in the egg and stir it through to make a moist
     mixture.

5.   Add the breadcrumbs and mix thoroughly so that the
     mixture binds together nicely. Use your hands to
     make 15 small meatballs.

6.   Heat the oil in a frying pan and gently cook the meat-
     balls, turning them until they're golden brown.

7.   Put them on a non-stick baking tray and cook them in
     the oven for 15 minutes.

8.   Serve 4–5 meatballs with a portion of brown rice and
     cover with the tomato sauce.

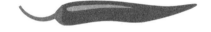

TOMATO SAUCE

Ingredients

1 tbsp olive oil

½ onion, finely chopped

2 garlic cloves, crushed

1 x 400g tin of chopped
   tomatoes

1 tsp cider vinegar

a pinch of sugar

a handful of chopped basil

pepper

**Va Va Voom
Factor**
Full of
anti-inflammatory
compounds, basil is also
a good source of
magnesium which relaxes
our muscles, improves
blood flow and is the
essential catalyst for
energy production.

Method

1. Heat the olive oil in a saucepan and cook the onions
    and garlic over a low heat until they are soft and
    transparent.

2. Add the chopped tomatoes, cider vinegar, sugar and
    a pinch of pepper, to taste.

3. Cook for about 5 minutes until the mixture thickens,
    then stir through the basil and cook for another
    minute before serving.

OVEN-BAKED VENISON SAUSAGES WITH SWEET POTATO MASH

Serves 2
Suitable for Intro and Cruising Days

Ingredients

4 venison sausages

2 medium sweet potatoes

1–2 tbsp olive oil

salt and pepper

Va Va Voom Factor

Venison is full of lean protein and is also an outstanding source of iron, containing double the amount per 100g than a steak.

Method

1. Preheat the oven to 190°C/170°C fan/gas mark 5.

2. Place the sausages on a baking tray and cook for 25–30 minutes, turning occasionally, until they're golden brown.

3. Peel and slice the sweet potatoes into quarters. Boil in salted water for about 20–25 minutes until they're soft.

4. Drain the potatoes and mash with the olive oil, using a potato masher. Season with salt and pepper and serve with the sausages.

GRILLED CHICKEN 3 WAYS

Serves 1
Suitable for Intro, Booster
and Cruising Days

GRILLED CHICKEN

Ingredients

1 chicken breast

tamari soy sauce

Va Va Voom Factor

A great source of lean protein, chicken is especially high in glutamine, which acts as fuel for the brain, and the branched-chain amino acids that increase endurance levels.

Method

1. Preheat the grill to high.

2. Open out the chicken breast and brush it with the tamari sauce.

3. Grill for about 7 minutes on each side or until golden and cooked through.

4. Add the chicken to one of the following three recipes.

1. WITH MIXED SALAD

Serves 1
Suitable for Intro, Booster
and Cruising Days

Ingredients

2 handfuls of rocket leaves

8 cherry tomatoes, halved

½ avocado, sliced

¼ cucumber, diced

1 tbsp roughly chopped coriander

French dressing (see page 222)

Va Va Voom Factor

Rocket is full of sulphur compounds which help to break down toxins in the liver. It's also packed with energy-boosting magnesium, B vitamins and iron.

Method

1.   Place all the vegetables in a salad bowl and scatter over the coriander.

2.   Pour over the dressing and toss it through the salad.

3.   Place the grilled chicken on top and serve.

2. WITH CAULIFLOWER RICE, SPINACH AND ROASTED RED VEGETABLES

Serves 1
Suitable for Intro, Booster and
Cruising Days

Va Va Voom Factor
Cauliflower is highly nutritious. It's especially high in vitamin C and full of so many other vitamins and minerals that it could almost power the electron transport chain by itself!

Ingredients

1 red pepper

garlic-infused olive oil

8 cherry tomatoes, on the vine

2 large handfuls of spinach leaves

½ a pouch of cauliflower rice (about 100g)

Method

1. Preheat the oven to 200°C/180°C fan/gas mark 6.

2. Slice the pepper into quarters, removing the seeds and the white flesh.

3. Flatten the pieces out and place in an ovenproof dish. Drizzle with olive oil and put in the oven for about 15 minutes, turning from time to time.

4. Brush the tomatoes with the olive oil and add to the peppers, cooking for another 10–15 minutes until they're soft and ready to serve.

5. Steam the spinach leaves for 3–4 minutes until they're wilted but still retain some form.

6. Meanwhile, microwave the cauliflower rice according to the instructions on the packet.

7. Place the chicken on a bed of cauliflower rice and surround with the rest of the vegetables.

3. WITH BROWN RICE AND STIR-FRIED VEGETABLES

Serves 1
Suitable for Intro, Booster and Cruising Days

Ingredients

1 tbsp sesame oil

a handful of sugar snap peas

2 spring onions, sliced diagonally

a handful of shredded cabbage

½ carrot, grated

a handful of beansprouts

½ garlic clove, crushed

3 chestnut mushrooms, sliced

tamari soy sauce

125g pre-cooked brown rice

Va Va Voom Factor

Cabbage is highly anti-inflammatory and full of fibre to balance your blood sugar, which could explain why some studies have shown it may reduce the risk of type 2 diabetes.

Method

1. Heat the oil in a frying pan and add the sugar snaps, spring onions, cabbage and carrot and cook for about 3 minutes over a low heat until the vegetables start to soften.

2. Add the beansprouts, garlic, mushrooms and the pre-cooked rice. Add the soy sauce and stir through the vegetable mixture so that it's fully coated.

3. Cook for another 2–3 minutes until the vegetables are tender but still retain their form.

4. Cut the grilled chicken into thick slices and lay on top of the vegetables and rice to serve.

SHEPHERD'S PIE WITH CRUSHED NEW POTATO TOPPING

Serves 4
Suitable for Intro and
Cruising Days

Ingredients

1kg new potatoes (with skin)

2 tbsp olive oil

1 tbsp rapeseed oil

600g lean minced lamb

3 carrots, sliced

2 garlic cloves, crushed

2 onions, finely chopped

2 x 400g tin of chopped tomatoes

1 tbsp tomato purée

1 lamb stock cube (making 200ml stock)

a few sprigs of fresh thyme

1 tsp Worcester sauce

salt and pepper

Va Va Voom Factor
The main fibre content of potatoes is in their skin, so new potatoes are the smart potato option if you want to keep your energy levels nice and stable. They're also a great everyday source of vitamin C and B6.

Method

1. Boil the new potatoes for about 20 minutes until soft, then strain, add the olive oil and roughly crush with a fork, so they still retain some form.

2. Heat the rapeseed oil in a large frying pan, add the mince and gently fry, turning regularly so that it browns evenly, then set aside on a plate.

3. Add the carrots, garlic and onions to the pan and gently fry until the carrots have softened and the onions are transparent but not brown.

4. Add the meat back to the pan along with the toma-
    toes, tomato purée and stock and mix well.

5. Add the thyme, season well with salt and pepper and
    a teaspoon of Worcester sauce.

6. Cook for about 20 minutes until the mixture has
    thickened.

7. In the meantime, preheat the oven to 190°C/170°C
    fan/gas mark 5.

8. Pour the mixture into an ovenproof dish and top with
    the crushed potato mixture.

9. Cook in the oven for about 25 minutes until the
    potato mixture has browned.

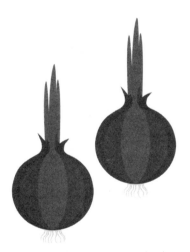

CHICKEN AND VEGETABLE CASSEROLE

Serves 4
Suitable for Intro and
Cruising Days

Va Va Voom Factor

Garlic is highly anti-inflammatory and contains sulphur compounds that play a big part in detoxifying the liver. It's also surprisingly high in vitamin C.

Ingredients

4 tbsp rapeseed oil

500g boneless, skinless chicken thighs

2 carrots

2 leeks

2 celery sticks

4 large garlic cloves, peeled

1 x 400g tin of butter beans, rinsed and drained

2 x 400g tin of chopped tomatoes

200g new potatoes, halved

a few sprigs of thyme

500ml chicken stock

salt and pepper

Method

1. Heat three tablespoons of rapeseed oil in a pan and brown the chicken thighs, turning from time to time.

2. In the meantime, slice the carrots lengthways into thick batons, cut the leeks into 2.5cm sections and slice the celery.

3. Remove the chicken from the pan and set aside. Add another tablespoon of oil if need be and add the carrots, leeks, celery and garlic cloves. Cover and sweat the vegetables over a low heat until they start to soften.

4.   Return the chicken to the pan along with the beans, tomatoes, potatoes and thyme. Season with salt and pepper.

5.   Add the chicken stock and bring to the boil, then turn down the heat and gently simmer for about 45 minutes until the meat is tender.

6.   Remove the sprigs of thyme before serving.

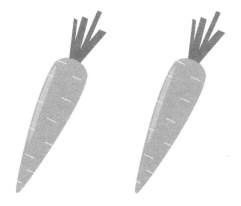

PRAWN AND PAK CHOI STIR FRY

Serves 2
Suitable for Intro, Booster
and Cruising Days

Va Va Voom Factor
Prawns are a great source of lean protein. They're also unusually high in copper and vitamin B12 which help to ward off anaemia.

Ingredients

200g pak choi

1 tbsp sesame oil

2 handfuls of sugar snap peas

3 spring onions, sliced diagonally

1 garlic clove, crushed

250g pre-cooked brown rice

100g beansprouts

150g cooked king prawns

2 tbsp tamari soy sauce

a handful of roughly chopped coriander

Method

1. Slice the woody end off the pak choi, slice the thicker white part of the leaf horizontally and cut the green leaf into long strips.

2. Heat the oil in a frying pan and add the sugar snap peas, spring onions and the white part of the pak choi. Cook over a low heat until the vegetables soften.

3. Stir through the garlic, rice and beansprouts and cook for another 2 minutes.

4. Add the prawns and the soy sauce, turning the mixture so that it's fully coated.

5.   Finally, add the rest of the pak choi and cook until it's slightly wilted but still retains its shape.

6.   Sprinkle each portion with fresh coriander before serving.

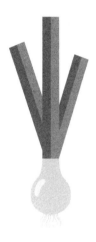

ROASTED HADDOCK WITH CITRUS RICE

Serves 2
Suitable for Intro, Booster
and Cruising Days

Ingredients

2½ tbsp olive oil

2 smoked haddock fillets
(skin on)

200g cherry tomatoes,
halved

2 tbsp pitted black olives,
halved

a handful of basil leaves

100g frozen garden peas

4 spring onions, sliced diagonally

120g green lentils

250g pre-cooked brown rice

juice of 1 lemon

a handful of coriander

salt and pepper

**Va Va
Voom Factor**
The high fibre
content of brown rice
helps to avoid blood
sugar spikes and keeps
you going for longer. It's
also packed with magne-
sium which is essential
for igniting the
process of energy
production.

Method

1. Preheat the oven to 200°C/180°C fan/gas mark 6.

2. Heat a tablespoon of oil in a frying pan and add the
    haddock fillets, skin side down. Cook for 2–3 minutes
    until the skin starts to become crisp.

3. Transfer the fish to an oven dish and cover with the
    tomatoes and olives. Add a pinch of salt and pepper
    and a drizzle of olive oil over the vegetables.

4.   Bake for about 15 minutes or until the fish is tender and the tomatoes cooked. Stir the basil through the tomatoes and olives.

5.   While the fish is cooking, add the peas to boiling water for 3 minutes, drain and set aside.

6.   Heat a tablespoon of olive oil in a frying pan and add the spring onions, cooking gently until soft.

7.   Add the peas, lentils and rice to the pan and cook for 1-2 minutes.

8.   Add the lemon juice, toss through the coriander and season with salt and pepper.

9.   Serve the fish on a bed of the rice mixture and top with the tomatoes and olives.

SARDINE FISHCAKES

Serves 2
Suitable for Intro and
Cruising Days

Va Va Voom Factor

Packed with protein, sardines are also an outstanding source of omega 3, keeping our heart and blood vessels in top working order and supporting cognitive function and mental performance.

Ingredients

300g potatoes

1 can of sardines in spring water

juice of ½ lemon

2 tbsp chopped parsley

a pinch of plain flour

1 tbsp rapeseed oil

Method

1. Boil the potatoes in water until they're soft. Drain and mash thoroughly.

2. Place the sardines in a bowl and break them into flakes with a fork.

3. Add the potato, lemon juice and parsley to the bowl and then mix thoroughly so that all the ingredients are evenly distributed.

4. Dust your hands with a little plain flour and mould the mixture into 4 fishcakes.

5. Heat the oil in a frying pan and gently fry the fishcakes for 3–4 minutes on each side until crispy and golden.

PAN-FRIED SALMON WITH GREEN LENTILS AND GARLIC-ROASTED VEGETABLES

Serves 2
Suitable for Intro, Booster and Cruising Days

Ingredients

1 tbsp rapeseed oil

2 salmon fillets (skin on)

1 x 400g tin of Puy lentils, rinsed and drained

Garlic-roasted vegetables (see page 264)

Va Va Voom Factor

Salmon is a top source of DHA, an omega 3 fatty acid which is essential for brain function and cognitive performance. It also helps improve circulation so that our cells receive sufficient oxygen to produce energy.

Method

1. Heat the oil in a frying pan.

2. Add the salmon fillets skin-side down and cook until the skin is crispy.

3. Turn the salmon over and cook for another 2 minutes or until cooked through. If the fillets are thick, you may need to cook each side for a minute as well.

4. Add the lentils to the pan for the last minute or so to warm them through.

5. Place the salmon on a bed of lentils and serve with the garlic-roasted vegetables.

GRILLED SALMON WITH STIR-FRIED VEGETABLES AND BROWN RICE

Serves 2
Suitable for Intro, Booster and
Cruising Days

Va Va Voom Factor
Baby corn provides a good dose of fibre which will provide sustained energy to keep you going. It also contains some iron and vitamin C.

Ingredients

2 salmon fillets

2½ tbsp tamari soy sauce

1 tbsp sesame oil

2 handfuls of baby corn

3 spring onions, sliced diagonally

2 handfuls of shredded cabbage

1 red pepper, deseeded and cut into strips

2 handfuls of beansprouts

½ garlic clove, crushed

6 chestnut mushrooms, sliced

250g pre-cooked brown rice

Method

1. Preheat the grill to high.

2. Brush the salmon fillets with soy sauce and place under the grill for about 8 minutes or until cooked through.

3. In the meantime, heat the oil in a frying pan and add the baby corn, spring onions, cabbage and peppers and cook for about 3 minutes over a low heat until the vegetables start to soften.

4. Add the beansprouts, garlic and mushrooms along with the pre-cooked rice. Stir the rest of the soy sauce through the mixture so that it's fully coated.

5. Cook for another 2–3 minutes until the vegetables are tender but still retain their form.

6. Divide the mixture between two plates and top with a salmon fillet.

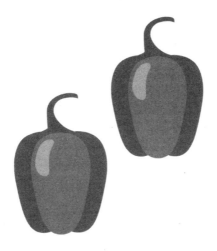

LENTIL AND VEGETABLE CASSEROLE

Serves 4
Suitable for Intro, Booster
and Cruising Days

Va Va Voom Factor
The combination of protein and fibre in lentils makes them an ideal food to balance blood sugar. They're also an excellent source of folate and iron.

Ingredients

1 red pepper

1 yellow pepper

2 large carrots

3 tbsp rapeseed oil

1 large leek, thickly sliced

3 garlic cloves

2 medium courgettes, thickly sliced

½ tsp paprika

½ tsp dried oregano

2 x 400g tin of chopped tomatoes

350ml vegetable stock

100g red lentils

2 x 250g pouches of pre-cooked quinoa

salt and pepper

Method

1. Deseed the peppers and cut into quarters. Cut the carrots lengthways into thick batons about 5cm long.

2. Heat the oil in a large pan and add the peppers, carrots, leek and garlic. Cover and sweat gently over a low heat for about 10 minutes, ensuring that they don't stick to the pan or start to colour.

3. Add the courgettes, paprika and oregano. Stir the vegetables thoroughly and continue to sweat for a further 5 minutes.

4.   Add the chopped tomatoes, stock and lentils. Season
     with salt and pepper and bring to the boil, then
     simmer for 25–30 minutes until the lentils are cooked
     through.

5.   Serve with 125g of pre-cooked quinoa per person.

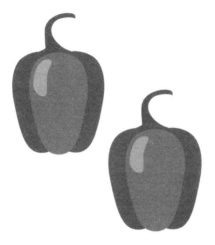

VEGETABLE AND BEAN CHILLI

Serves 4
Suitable for Intro and
Cruising Days

Ingredients

1 medium sweet potato

¾ tsp cumin

¾ tsp cayenne pepper

¾ tsp cinnamon

1½ tbsp olive oil

1 onion, finely chopped

2 garlic cloves, crushed

1 red pepper, deseeded and
  sliced into squares

1 medium courgette, cut into
  2.5cm chunks

1 red chilli, deseeded and finely sliced

1 green chilli, deseeded and finely sliced

1 x 400g tin of kidney beans

1 x 400g tin of chopped tomatoes

1 tbsp tomato purée

a handful of finely chopped coriander

2 x 250g pouches of pre-cooked brown rice (optional)

Va Va Voom Factor

Chillies contain an anti-inflammatory compound called capsaicin which gives them their spicy taste. The perceived heat from the capsaicin can trick your brain into responding by desensitising our sensory receptors, which can help to reduce and relieve the draining impact of long-term pain.

Method

1.   Preheat the oven to 200°C/180°C fan/gas mark 6.

2.   Scrub the sweet potato thoroughly, cut into 2.5cm chunks and place on a baking sheet.

3.   Mix a pinch of cumin, cayenne pepper and cinnamon with a teaspoon of olive oil and pour over the sweet potato, making sure it's evenly coated.

4.   Bake for about 30 minutes or until cooked through.

5.   Meanwhile, heat the rest of the oil in a large frying pan and cook the onion, garlic and red pepper over a low heat until they're soft.

6.   Add in the courgette and chillies and stir through.

7.   Add half a teaspoon of cumin, cayenne pepper and cinnamon to the pan and cook for 5–10 minutes.

8.   Drain and rinse the kidney beans and then add to the pan with the chopped tomatoes, tomato purée and half the coriander. If the mixture is too thick, add a small amount of water to loosen it.

9.   Bring to the boil and then gently simmer for 30 minutes.

10. Add the sweet potato and cook for 5 minutes. Serve with optional brown rice and scatter over the remaining coriander.

QUINOA, COURGETTE AND GOAT'S CHEESE-STUFFED PEPPERS

Serves 1
Suitable for Intro and
Cruising Days

Ingredients

30g quinoa

1 vegetable stock cube

1 tbsp rapeseed oil

50g courgettes, diced

½ small onion, finely chopped

1 garlic clove, crushed

6 cherry tomatoes, cut into
   quarters

2 red peppers

1 tbsp chopped parsley

15g goat's cheese

Va Va Voom factor

Parsley is more than just a garnish: it's a highly concentrated source of vitamin C, which is essential for the citric acid energy cycle. Gram for gram, it has 3 times as much vitamin C as an orange and a red pepper has twice as much. This dish is vitamin C city!

Method

1. Rinse the quinoa in cold water and then add to a saucepan. Cook the quinoa in double the amount of water with the stock cube for about 20 minutes or until the grains have softened and opened up.

2. While the quinoa is cooking, heat the oil in a frying pan and add the courgette, onion, garlic and tomatoes.

3. Cook gently for 10 minutes or until the vegetables have softened and then set aside on a plate.

4. When the quinoa is ready, strain it through a sieve and set aside.

5. Preheat the oven to 200°C/180°C fan/gas mark 6.

6. Slice the top off the peppers and carefully trim the white flesh inside, removing the core and the seeds, so that you have a clean, smooth interior.

7. Cook the peppers in the microwave on a high setting for 3 minutes so that they are soft and wilting but the structure hasn't collapsed.

8. In a bowl, mix together the cooked vegetables, quinoa and parsley and spoon it carefully into the peppers. Top each pepper with goat's cheese.

9. Cook in the oven for 15 minutes, and serve.

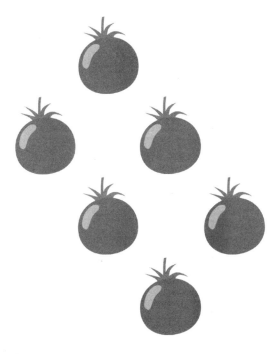

GARLIC-ROASTED VEGETABLES WITH (OPTIONAL) QUINOA

Serves 2
Suitable for Intro, Booster,
Cleansing and Cruising Days

Va Va Voom Factor
Butternut squash is full of carotenoids – powerful antioxidants which reduce inflammation and support heart function. It's also a very rounded source of the B vitamins we need for energy production.

Ingredients

2 red onions, cut into quarters

2 large carrots, cut lengthways into quarters

2 large courgettes, cut into chunks

2 red peppers, cut into chunks

100g butternut squash, cut into 2cm chunks

4 garlic cloves, unpeeled

1 tbsp chopped rosemary

2 tbsp olive oil

250g pre-cooked quinoa (not for Cleansing Days)

salt and pepper

Method

1.   Preheat the oven to 220°C/200°C fan/gas mark 7.

2.   Put all the vegetables and the garlic into a roasting tin.

3.   Add the rosemary to a tablespoon of olive oil and pour over the vegetables, mixing thoroughly with your hands to make sure they're properly coated with oil.

4.   Roast for 20–25 minutes until the vegetables are cooked through.

5. Remove the garlic cloves and squeeze out the soft garlic. Mix it with a tablespoon of olive oil and dot over the vegetables.

6. Serve with or without quinoa, depending on the phase of the plan you're in.

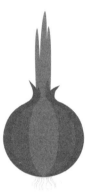

ROOT VEGETABLE MASH

Serves 2
Suitable for Intro, Booster
and Cruising Days

Ingredients

1 small swede

2 large carrots

1 large parsnip

1–2 tbsp olive oil

salt and pepper

NB: aim for about 1kg of
vegetables

Va Va Voom Factor

Rich in complex carbohydrate, starchy parsnips and swede provide a quick win in energy terms that won't burn out too soon. This is a sustaining side dish that will keep you going nicely.

Method

1. Peel the vegetables and cut them into chunks.

2. Boil in salted water for about 20–25 minutes until they're soft.

3. Drain the vegetables and mash with the olive oil, using a potato masher. Season with salt and pepper.

SWEET POTATO FRIES

Serves 1
Suitable for Intro and
Cruising Days

Ingredients

100g sweet potato

1 tsp rapeseed oil

a pinch of paprika, cayenne
   pepper or chilli powder
   (optional)

salt and pepper

Va Va Voom Factor
Sweet potatoes are a great alternative to standard potatoes because they cause a lower spike in blood sugar. The high fibre content will keep you going for longer and the skin is full of energy-boosting B vitamins, iron and copper.

Method

1. Preheat the oven to 200°C/180°C fan/gas mark 6.

2. Scrub the sweet potato thoroughly, cut lengthways into wedges and place on a baking tray. Mix with the oil until thoroughly coated. Add the paprika, cayenne pepper or chilli powder if you want a little bit of spice.

3. Season with salt and pepper and bake for about 20 minutes until crispy and golden.

Snacks

Smart snacking is essential for supporting your Va Va Voom throughout the day. If you leave several hours between meals, your blood sugar will drop, you'll start to flag and you'll feel absolutely desperate for a quick energy fix. This means your hormones will be in charge of your food choices instead of your brain and you're likely to reach for certain Va Va Voom robbers to keep you going. A balanced snack in the afternoon that combines protein and fibre will help to break up the long gap between lunch and dinner and keep your Va Va Voom levels on track.

Make sure you respect the portion guidelines for your snacks so you don't end up eating 5 meals a day! If you don't feel hungry between meals, you don't have to force yourself to have a snack. Not everyone will feel the need for a snack as some people have a more sensitive glucose response than others; as long as your energy levels are stable and you're not craving sugary food or refined carbohydrate, it's fine to wait until the next meal.

SPICY ROASTED CHICKPEAS

*Makes about 25 servings
(15g per serving)
Suitable for Intro, Booster
and Cruising Days*

**Va
Va Voom
Factor**
Packed with fibre and
protein, chickpeas are a
perfectly balanced snack
which will keep your
energy levels nicely
topped up. They're also
a great plant source
of iron and
zinc.

Ingredients

1 x 400g tin of chickpeas

1 tsp olive oil

a pinch of garam masala or
cayenne pepper

salt and pepper

Method

1. Preheat the oven to 180°C /160°C fan/gas mark 4.

2. Rinse the chickpeas and pat dry, discarding any skins
that have come off.

3. Drizzle with olive oil, add a generous pinch of your
chosen spice and mix thoroughly, ensuring the chickpeas are properly coated. Don't overdo the oil or they
may go soggy!

4. Season well with salt and pepper and lay them out on
a baking tray.

5. Cook for 45 minutes or until the chickpeas are nicely crispy,
turning from time to time so that they're evenly cooked.

6. Serve out a 15g portion for a snack. Store the rest in
an airtight container.

ROSEMARY-ROASTED ALMONDS

Makes 15 servings (7–8 almonds per serving)
Suitable for Intro, Booster, Cleansing and Cruising Days

Ingredients

150g unsalted almonds

2–3 sprigs of rosemary

1–2 tbsp olive oil

2 tbsp finely chopped rosemary

salt and pepper

Va Va Voom Factor

A triple whammy of Va Va Voom here – almonds are packed with magnesium, which starts our energy engine; they help to reduce blood sugar levels; and they support heart and circulatory health by lowering cholesterol.

Method

1. Preheat the oven to 180°C/160°C fan/gas mark 4.

2. Place the nuts on a baking tray with the sprigs of rosemary and cook for 10–15 minutes until the nuts are brown but not burnt.

3. Add the olive oil and chopped rosemary to a bowl and stir together.

4. Remove the nuts from the oven, season with salt and pepper and toss with the rosemary oil mixture so that they're thoroughly coated.

5. Serve out a portion of 7–8 almonds for a snack to have with a piece of fruit. Store the rest in an airtight container.

Acknowledgements

When my agent, Barbara Levy, asked me about the most common health issues in my nutrition clinic, low energy sprang to mind immediately and so the idea for Va Va Voom was conceived. Her enthusiasm and support for this project has made it possible for me to turn that initial concept into this beautiful book.

Special thanks are due to all the team at Headline Home who have worked so hard to develop and promote this book. I'm particularly grateful to Muna Reyal for spotting the potential of the concept and her guidance throughout the process has been both invaluable and inspirational; to Kate Miles, who's been exceptionally patient and good-humoured as we grappled with the best way to present all the Va Va Voom information; to Siobhan Hooper, who instinctively understood my vague feedback and weaved her magic on the design to make it a thing of beauty and to Sophie Elletson, for carefully checking every last detail. You've all been incredibly helpful and professional and it's been a pleasure to work with you.

The dedication of my Va Va Voom guinea pigs has been second to none and they have applied themselves to the plan with enormous enthusiasm and excellent results. Huge thanks to my brother Rob and my sister-in-law Rosemary Lynch and to Sarah Walker for working with me on this. Your feedback (which was robust at times!) has been a great help and I know you're benefitting from the extra Va Va Voom.

There's nothing like a shared approach and my family do so love to get involved! As always, they've been consistently engaged and helpful throughout this project in many different ways. A shared flash of inspiration with my sister, Frankie Laws, led to the choice of Va Va Voom as a title. Very few family members have escaped my recipe testing but special thanks to my Dad, Frank Lynch, and my niece, Georgie Lynch, for bravely enduring my spicy turkey meatballs at our bank holiday picnic. Thanks also to my nephew, Ben Lynch, for our in-depth smoothie discussions, and to Catherine and Joe Laws, whose questions and comments have made me think harder about how to explain some of the Va Va Voom guidelines and principles.

And to my lovely friends who observed me locking myself away for 7 weeks to write this book and who quietly made sure I got the occasional break by planning some fabulous outings – Sue, Fiona, Dan, thanks for looking out for me.

Index

RECIPE INDEX